D0442552

Midlife Man

Art Hister, M.D.

Midlife Man

A not-so-threatening

guide to health and sex

for man at his peak

GREYSTONE BOOKS
DOUGLAS & MCINTYRE
VANCOUVER/TORONTO

Copyright © 1998 by Art Hister

98 99 00 01 02   5 4 3 2 1

All rights reserved. No part of this book may be reproduced, stored in a retrieval system or transmitted in any form or by any means without the prior permission of the publisher or, in the case of photocopying or other reprographic copying, a licence from CANCOPY (Canadian Reprography Collective), Toronto, Ontario.

Greystone Books
A division of Douglas & McIntyre Ltd.
1615 Venables Street
Vancouver, British Columbia
V5L 2H1

CANADIAN CATALOGUING IN PUBLICATION DATA
Hister, Art
   Midlife man

ISBN 1-55054-656-2

1. Climacteric, Male.   I. Title.
RC884.H57 1998   616.6'93   C98-910793-0

Every attempt has been made to trace accurate ownership of copyrighted material in this book. Errors and omissions will be corrected in subsequent editions, provided that notification is sent to the publisher.

The following copyright holders have given permission to use quoted material:
From Ogden Nash, *Many Long Years Ago*, reprinted by permission of Little, Brown and Company. From "Midlife Myths" by Winifred Gallagher, *The Atlantic Monthly*, May 1993. Reprinted by permission of Winifred Gallagher. From *Male Menopause*, excerpt © 1992 by Jed Diamond. Reprinted by permission of Sourcebooks, Inc. From "Tower Of Song," words and music by Leonard Cohen. Copyright © 1991 Sony/ATV Songs LLC. All rights administered by Sony/ATV Music Publishing, 8 Music Square West, Nashville, TN 37203. All rights reserved. Used by permission. From "Father's Little Helper" by Maureen Dowd, *The New York Times*, April 26, 1998. Copyright © 1998 by *The New York Times*. Reprinted by permission. From "Endocrine Factors in Geriatric Sexuality" by John E. Morley, *Clinics in Geriatric Medicine* 7, February 1991. Reprinted by permission of John E. Morley. From "Big Yellow Taxi," words and music by Joni Mitchell. Copyright © 1970 Crazy Crow Music (Renewed). All rights administered by Sony/ATV Music Publishing, 8 Music Square West, Nashville, TN 37203. All rights reserved. Used by permission.

Editing by Nancy Flight
Jacket design by Peter Cocking
Front jacket photograph by Chick Rice
Text design by Val Speidel
Typesetting by Brenda and Neil West, BN Typographics West, and Val Speidel
Illustrations by Marian Bantjes
Printed and bound in Canada by Friesens

The publisher gratefully acknowledges the support of the Canada Council for the Arts and the British Columbia Ministry of Tourism, Small Business and Culture. The publisher also acknowledges the financial support of the Government of Canada through the Book Publishing Industry Development Program for its publishing activities..

For Phyllis, Jonah, and Tim

Contents

Preface

It is, of course, impossible to write any book without a great deal of help, and in this case, I needed more than my fair share.

The idea for this book originated with Rob Sanders, whose optimistic nature has never failed to impress me. As she was last time, my editor, Nancy Flight, was a delight to work with, and although in my opinion, she again left much of my best material on the cutting-room floor, I must reluctantly admit that she did improve the text considerably. Thanks even to Robin Van Heck, who cut still more.

As always, my family offered me more love and support than I probably deserve. Even better, they have given me permission to make as much fun of them as I feel necessary, although I am still not sure I will allow them to see a copy of this book. Several friends and relatives— KM, Hanty Sherry and the Dean, Bri-Bri, Mary Ann, Jenny, Norman, Jeannie, Sarah B., Pat, and Leonard—also deserve special mention for having put up with all that whining for all those months, not that it isn't gonna start up again very soon.

The physicians and other health professionals who offered me invaluable assistance and advice—even though they did not always agree with my views, and who, I hasten to add, are not responsible for any of the editorial opinions—include Dr. Ray Baker, Dr. Susan Barr, Dr. Rosemary Basson, Dr. Richard Bebb, Dr. Vicki Bernstein, Dr. Howard Fenster, Dr. John Fleetham, Dr. Jon Fleming, Dr. Brad Fritz, Dr. Martin Gleave, Dr. Laurie Halparin, Dr. Theresa Hogarth, Dr. David Kendler, Dr. James McCormack, Dr. John Morley, Dr. Robert Rangno, Dr. Oliver Robinow, Dr. Simon Pimstone, Dr. David Thompson, and Dr. John Wade. Every one of these folks is the kind of doctor you should be lucky enough to have as your own.

I must also add that nearly every one of these people—I lie, it was really every one—asked me to promise that I would mention that they are not in any way responsible for any of the humour in the text (or lack of it), and several of them also asked me to note that they had tried as hard as they could to dissuade me from using some of the jokes that I did eventually include. It's clearly not easy trying to be funny in this country, especially among doctors.

I must say a few more words about my use of humour. I have always used humour to communicate, not only with the public but especially with my family and friends. I know no other way. And in my medical life, especially in my writing and broadcasting, I have found that humour allows me to deal with issues that are often very difficult to discuss. Believe me, it's not easy doing an open-line show about rectal problems on Sunday morning, but humour gets me through. Medical information can be so daunting, and medical people can be so intimidating, that a lay person is often frightened to even ask questions about his or her condition. For me, humour has always been a way around those barriers.

But in using humour, I am also cognizant of two important things. First, I realize that lots of people do not agree with me, and they believe that to laugh at something serious is to mock it. So let me say this very plainly: when I joke about a medical condition, and especially about a person who has a symptom or a disease, I do not intend the slightest bit of disrespect towards that person. Making fun is not making light. After nearly thirty years as a family physician, I know how hard it is to deal with many of these issues and how lonely it sometimes seems when the world does not appreciate the difficulties you may be encountering. I have always said, and I very much believe, that I have learned much more from my patients than I have ever taught them. It's just that I also believe that you have to be able to laugh at yourself and your problem (within reason, of course), or else the battle is lost.

Second, humour is like pizza. Everyone has his or her own idea of the best topping, and one man's irreplaceable anchovy-feta-sausage-onion selection (how does my son sleep after eating something like that?) is the next man's inedible concoction. So if you are insulted by anything I say in this book, take solace from the fact that you are not alone. I am an equal-opportunity insulter, but I make more fun of myself (actually I make most fun of my wife) than I do of others. To borrow a bit from Tom Lehrer, "If Hister's arse can take it, so can you."

As to the topics covered in the text, careful readers will note that I have been selective. I have not, for example, discussed any cancers except for prostate cancer and a very brief bit about colon and rectal cancer. Space left me little choice, but I also feel strongly that anyone with a chronic health problem such as cancer should consult a book specifically dedicated to that problem.

Introduction

Middle age is when you're sitting at home on a Saturday night and
the telephone rings and you hope it's not for you.

—Ogden Nash

There are probably as many myths about midlife now as there
were about aging thirty years ago.

—Gilbert Brim, quoted in "Midlife Myths" by Winifred Gallagher, *Atlantic Monthly*

I'm still not sure how the single-celled idea to write a book that was
originally supposed to be titled something like *The Crumbling, Aging
Male—A First-Person Perspective* came to life. But when I told my wife
of this vague proposal from my publisher, she immediately said, "I
can't think of anyone who would be more right to do such a book than
you, dear."

Sadly, my wife was far from a lone voice. Nearly all my colleagues,
most listeners to my radio show, my car mechanic, my lawyer, strang-
ers I met in bars, indeed just about everyone who knows me at all, and
some who knew me only for minutes, seemed to instantly agree that
yes, I would indeed be the perfect person to write a book about "how
all you guys deteriorate as you get older," as an ex-friend of mine put
it, not even bothering to suppress her smirk.

This idea, then, seemed to have "legs" right from the moment it
first saw light. The clincher, however, was my teenage sons' regular
and terribly insensitive reminders that even though I had once worked
at a free clinic and even though I had truly, honestly swear-to-God
been at Woodstock (the original one, not the twenty-fifth anniversary

ersatz one with all those balding, wrinkled, potbellied has-beens—both performers and attendees), I have indeed become, as my boys like to say, "like really old, man." So even though my thirty-year-old bell-bottoms did eventually come back into style (though clearly not on me), everyone's snide remarks finally led me to acknowledge that my days as a boy-wonder (a legend in my own mind) had indeed come and gone. I have been forced to recognize that I am well into the next phase of my life, a recognition shoved in my face recently when, along with twenty thousand others of my generation, I attended a Van Morrison–Joni Mitchell–Bob Dylan last-hurrah concert. Now that I have become a committed middle-aged nonsmoker, when it came time for the audience to wave its lighters during a particularly nostalgic number, I waved my cellular phone instead. And so did most of the people around me.

"So why not write about it," I asked myself. "Especially since the publisher has been dumb enough to give me an advance, meagre though it is." Besides, I reasoned further, maybe I have a duty to write this book, to let my fellow aging brothers, and especially their spouses and inheritors, know that at the age of fifty, a male is not necessarily so close to death that he can feel her hot breath on his neck.

Having seen this milestone come and go, I have become convinced that a man at fifty is still quite young. And because of medical advances, as well as the fact that those of us now entering our sixth decade have by and large lived a much healthier life than our fathers did, many more of us near-geezers will live into our eighties and nineties than ever before, a thought that no doubt terrifies our inheritors. And they may have a bit of a point because God only knows how society will handle a world overrun with shrivelled, slippered, unshaven, leaky ninety-year-old men. For a start, they're going to have to build a lot more sit-down spaces and bathrooms in the malls. At that Morrison–Mitchell–Dylan concert, for example, the lineups in the men's washrooms were out the door, as all the old farts seemed to take forever to get their business done.

This book, then, is about middle age in a male: his fantasies, his fears, his failures, his frustrations, his physical falloff, his finagling, and his future, and my purpose is to let every man over forty know what to expect as he plunges into the coming two decades. But because I have learned over the years that the average guy would rather bring Andrea Dworkin or Roseanne home to meet his mom and dad than admit that he wants or needs to find out more about his health, I also intend this book to be read by women who live with, work with, or deal with men. Not only do I hope this book will help such women understand what is happening to old lifeless lard-butt, who prefers to sit in his living room soaking up the suds rather than to sit on his cycle sweating off the suet, but I also hope that many women will read appropriate sections of this text aloud to their mates or male colleagues and thus perhaps prompt them to read it on their own, and maybe even goad them into doing something with the information.

"But," many of you are probably wondering, "aside from your need to write it and your wish to make a few extra bucks, Art, why is a book like this really necessary? After all, we have all those health shows on television and radio to tell us about this stuff."

Over the last few years we have indeed witnessed a rapidly growing interest in health and a corresponding explosion of investigative programs as well as open-mouth television and radio shows (one of which I host, by the way—consult your local listings for the time in your area, and if you can't find a listing, bug your local station to pick up this excellent show) to cater to this interest. The problem, however, is that such programs, governed as they all are by the ratings they draw and little else, are by their very nature both superficial and sensation seeking. So if, for example, you would like to know how and why so many left-handed cross-dressing transsexuals have murdered their lesbian lovers in midlife, television will undoubtedly be happy to provide you with the answer, and I'm sure it has already done so. But if you would like to know in some depth what happens to normal middle-aged men (not an oxymoron, by the way), there is little reliable, verifiable, and accessible information available to you, and much of what is available is often more myth or wishful thinking than reality.

This paucity of information about middle-aged men stands in stark contrast to what we know about women and middle age. As anyone with an interest in health can attest, these days women approaching menopause are the medical, social, cultural, political, even economic flavour du jour. Consequently, we are all deluged daily with data about menopause-related changes, what choices women can make to ease this passage, how long they will suffer with the symptoms, and how they are likely to fare. Every day, it seems, spawns yet another article or a new finding about menopause, which is why a typical man probably knows more about what estrogen can do for hot flushes and vaginal dryness than he does about what finasteride can do for his swollen prostate.

Now please note that I am not at all blaming menopausal women for this disparity, mostly because, for personal reasons, I would never dare do that. I value my well-being, and my place in bed. It's not women's fault that men have so little information about themselves. No, the fault for that, I'm afraid, resides nearly entirely with men themselves. The sad truth is that in the past, most men, but especially younger ones, were clearly not much interested in their bodies, particularly in its failings.

To be fair, the reason for this lack of concern about health matters stems from the average younger man's generally happy physiological state, because if he is born healthy and he can avoid getting into accidents and developing chronic illnesses, very little generally goes wrong to disturb the average under-forty-year-old man's normal condition of intact wellness and his corresponding state of blissful and willful medical ignorance.

So while from a rather early age on, women are constantly reminded of their oh-so-changeable bodies—periods, PMS, pregnancies, parturition, postpartum pits—a typically clueless and average man can swing along from the time he starts to shave until the time he is getting up twice a night to pee and never notice a change in how his body functions. In addition, when a medical problem does crop up, the typical male reacts in one of two ways. He tends either to deny that there is anything wrong until it can no longer be avoided ("You know, George, you really should have come to see me before this lump got to be the size of a grapefruit." "I know, Doc, only I was sure it would go away on its own") or else he panics and immediately presumes the worst. To most men, nearly every cough represents a budding pneumonia and every two-day headache heralds a brain tumour, until proven otherwise. Happily, such proof can generally be offered in short order by a wife who says, "Grow up. It's only a cold." The physiological constancy of their bodies married to men's natural aversion to knowing more about their health bred an understandable medical nonchalance and lack of curiosity in the men who came before my generation.

Science obliged men who did not want to know more by not doing much research on the normal events that happen to healthy men. Thus, we know a great deal about old men; we know a great deal about boys;

we know the most about sick men. But we really don't know much about what normal, middle-aged men should expect or do.

Things are changing, however. Prompted by the example of baby-boomer women, who have prodded and persuaded the medical world to find answers for what is happening to their bodies at every stage of their lives—from the time they are fetuses in utero, when they first begin to move their jaws way more than their male counterparts do (it's true, and I am smart enough and scared enough to make no editorial comment about that) to the time they finally rejoin their husbands, who predeceased them, in happy eternal interment—many male members of the most narcissistic, self-involved generation to have ever come along (until Generation X got here, of course; now there is a bunch of crybabies sans peer) have also taken an increasing interest in their bodies. These men have begun to bleat loudly, as only baby boomers can do, that they want answers about what is happening to them right now, what is likely to happen to them in the near future, and what they can do about stopping it.

To silence those lambs, I am happy to say that we are now seeing an increasing amount of attention paid to the health concerns of normal midlife men, especially to what some researchers call andropause or viropause, the so-called male menopause. We have also witnessed a corresponding outpouring of headline-grabbing findings about this newly discovered and seemingly inevitable passage in every man's life.

As always, though, the headlines don't tell the whole story. Is there really reliable evidence that a universal and inevitable metabolic or hormonal change affects all men at a certain time in life? And what about the infamous "male midlife crisis," a rather indistinct term referring to a cataclysmic event that presumably stems from ennui or fear. Is a midlife crisis really inevitable, or is it simply the product of some overeager Hollywood scriptwriters' imaginations? Is every wife doomed to wake up one day to find her trusty five-year-old, seven-seater Dodge van replaced by a two-seater silver Porsche in her driveway? (And who is most likely to occupy that second seat?) Or worse, is every Brittany and Chelsea and Tiffany a potential stepmom to every menopausal Mary's or Jan's or Linda's kids? Should every aging libidinally challenged man start taking testosterone as hormone-replacement therapy? Should his spouse do the same? And what about Viagra? Is it really the answer to all your drooping dreams? Are

Viagrified men the new Godzillas—hairy, fearsome, and on the prowl? You'll have to read on to find out, I'm afraid.

But one last word before you do. If you are looking for cheap jokes and sad endings, you will be disappointed. The cheap jokes are here in abundance, of course. I'm a Jewish Canadian male, after all. That's the only way we know how to survive.

The sad ending, however, is not here. You see, I strongly disagree with those authors, the newly minted minions of male menopause mavens, who claim that despite their outward bravado, nearly all middle-aged men are silently unhappy creatures, terrified of losing their youth and petrified of old age. I do not agree, as so many authors seem to claim, that most middle-aged men are desperate to find a way out of their caught-in-the-middle position (no longer man-on-the-way-up, not yet man-on-the-way-out), frantically seeking equally unhappy brothers with whom they can go into the woods, wrestle in the mud, cry together over a few beers or herbal tea, and beat some drums.

Rather, I believe that middle age is a great time of life, a time when most of us, men and women both, finally feel as if we're on top of whatever hill we had set out to climb so many years ago (or at least as close to the top as we're ever likely to get, given how out of breath many of us become these days when we do any climbing). I also believe that middle age is that time of life when we are most flexible and most able to roll with the punches life inevitably hits us with. Middle age is when we are most able to accommodate those changes that will allow us to be what we want to be when we finally grow up.

I believe that for many men, probably most men, what happens to us in midlife is not nearly as unwelcome as we have been led to believe. For most of us, midlife is the best time of life, and many of the changes that accompany middle age are not only pleasant but the harbingers of even better things to come.

So be warned by a man who owns a ten-year-old Mazda MPV seven-seater van (I'm probably too fat to fit comfortably into a small sports car, my bad back won't let me bend that far, and besides, for a Jewish man, there are way too many gears in those vroom boxes). Middle age is not the beginning of the end. Most men come through their middle years happy with themselves and with their lives, proud of their achievements, valued by their families and society in general, and determined to make the second half of their lives even better and richer. Although I must ruefully acknowledge, as most of my peers must too, that many of the goals I had set myself in my younger years will never be achieved (I will never figure out how a carburetor works or even what it is, I will never ski a double-black-diamond run—in fact, I may never even get down a blue run in one schuss—and I will certainly never play the piano for the symphony, in part because I will probably never even learn to play the piano unless I take a few lessons), I also believe that in many other very important respects, for me and for most midlife men, the present is pleasant, perhaps even the best there is, and the next few years promise to be just as good.

CHAPTER 1

That Was Then—
This Is Now

If youth's theme is potential, midlife's is reality: childhood fantasies are
past, the fond remembrances of age are yet to be, and the focus is on
coming to terms with the finite resources of the here and now. The
overwhelming majority . . . accomplish this developmental task . . .
through a long, gentle process. . . .

—WINIFRED GALLAGHER, "Midlife Myths," *Atlantic Monthly*

Midlife is the black box of human development. . . .

—DR. ORVILLE GILBERT BRIM,
Director of the MacArthur Foundation Research Network
on Successful Midlife Development

There was a time, I remember, when my hair did not plug up the drain
after a shower, when my knees did not make those high-pitched,
loose-board creaks they now emit every morning as I take my first
steps, when I needed only one pair of unifocal glasses, when the pain
from even a severely pulled muscle lasted no more than a few days and
required no more therapy than my old standby typical-male remedy of
feeling extremely sorry for myself, and when I didn't hesitate to bend
down to pick up an object on the ground or help a friend move his
household goods or try to open the lid of a virgin pickle jar using only
my still-firm hands.

I also remember when I could eat huge quantities of food and lie
down immediately afterwards without worrying about how this activity would affect my belt line or how far up the esophagus my overly
active digestive juices would burn. Back in those days, I could still

devour mounds and mounds of several kinds of garlic sausage, the amount limited only by my consideration for the company I would have to face following the meal, and I could still drink as much alcohol as I could afford to buy or, better yet, have bought for me.

These days I'm a changed man. My ever receding hairline has retreated to what I know is (alas!) a temporary trench on the top of my skull. At the same time, perhaps as some perverse form of compensation, there are now many new tufts of hair protruding from previously nonhairy portals to my body. I wear trifocal glasses, and even then I can't read very well unless the page is held at exactly the right distance from my eyes. My back emits at least one sharp stab of pain and often several if I turn around or bend over without due caution, my belt line has slipped below my midriff and now lies within gearing-down distance of my knees, my constant and most trusted companion is a bottle of extra-strength, double-duty antacid tablets, and perhaps most troublesome, I have to think very carefully about how much and what kind of liquids I consume before going to a movie or getting on a plane in case I don't get an aisle seat and my prostate gland turns uncooperative. For a fifty-year-old man, hell is a window seat in economy class next to Leona Helmsley on a plane delayed on takeoff.

Moreover, gravity's unfettered run at re-exerting its control on my naïve tissues has led most of my external parts, as well as a few internal ones, to slither south. Worse, some of me has also started to shrink, and since I'm only five foot six, I don't really have that much to give back. Worst of all, much of me has begun to deteriorate. As an added indignity, some of my parts have even started to hurt occasionally without any evident provocation. When provoked, they hurt even more.

So what has happened to me? Without realizing it, without expecting it, and certainly without welcoming it, I have become my father: balding, bulging, buckling, belching, and middle-aged. It's gone so far that I have even considered buying a recliner (last year, 45 per cent of recliners sold in the U.S. were bought by people between the ages of thirty-four and fifty-two) and going on a cruise. I have (I sheepishly admit) secretly studied brochures extolling the beauties of "Florida in the Winter," and—horrors!—I once even wore long underwear on what threatened to be a cool day—in July.

But in my generation I am certainly not an exception. All of us middle-agers are suffering these bodily insults and alarming symptoms of premature old foginess. Most guys I know have become quite altered —physically, emotionally, and spiritually—in the last few years.

This is nothing new. Similar changes happened to our fathers, to their fathers, and to all the fathers that came before them. What is new, however, is that an increasing number of us middle-aged gents want to know what these changes portend. Which ones are normal? Which changes are warning signals of impending physical or emotional disaster? What can we do about them? How can we prevent them? Where can we run to? And where can we hide?

The difficulty with answering these questions, however, is that in men, midlife is still a largely unstudied period of life. It has been claimed that we men are about twenty years behind our female counterparts in what science can tell us about what is normal in middle age. Happily, this state of affairs is rapidly changing, and men's midlife hormonal, psychological, and emotional changes are now the subjects of many studies. Until those studies are completed, however, we are left with much speculation, and as anyone can tell from the scads of books and articles that have recently appeared on middle age in men and that have come to significantly different conclusions, it is pretty easy to claim just about anything without having the necessary proof. That does not apply to what I am about to tell you, of course.

HEAVENS! A MALE MENOPAUSE?

About the only comfort all the other guys my age and I can draw from the many changes we have endured is the knowledge that they are not confined to men. Middle-aged women also undergo profound physical changes, but happily for them, women can at least attribute many of their symptoms to a defined, measurable, universally recognized, and treatable hormonal change: menopause. Thus, women who choose to can also make a good part of their midlife journey much less bumpy by hopping a ride on the Concorde of hormone therapy, which can at the very least dull or temper many of their more bothersome midlife symptoms.

What is not generally known is that many of us men suffer many of the same outrageous slings and symptoms that affect women going through menopause (no, men don't get vaginal dryness, but many of us do suffer from mood swings, increased anxiety, back pain, insomnia, headaches, and even hot flushes). Science has still not established, however, that in midlife men these symptoms are produced by hormonal changes, nor that a drop in hormone levels with age has much effect on men.

On one level, then, that makes the issue of whether men suffer a menopause rather cut-and-dried. If we adopt a narrow "medical" definition of menopause (and one that most lay people would accept as well) as simply "the cessation of menstruation, and by extension, the cessation of (these days we have to add "natural") reproductive ability," men clearly do not go through a male equivalent of menopause. So although a man's reproductive capacity diminishes somewhat with age, as so many men from our biblical forefathers Jacob and Abraham to Pablo Picasso and Tony Randall have exuberantly and visibly demonstrated, a man's ability to impregnate a partner can stay intact until old age, and as abhorrent as the thought may be to most of us, some very old men can and do sire inheritors. At least that's the story their much younger wives inevitably tell them. I mean, without DNA testing, who knows who Isaac's father really was?

But such a narrow definition of menopause drastically misses the mark I think, because for women, menopause is much more than a time when hormone levels drop and periods peter out and birth control ceases to be a worry. The several years that make up the perimenopausal and menopausal period are also a time of great upheaval and change—physical, emotional, psychological, economic, and spiritual—in almost every woman's life, a time when so much more than just her reproductive abilities are altered.

Middle-aged men experience most of these changes too. Most noticeably, our bodies change significantly, and these changes are visible not only to ourselves but to anyone lucky enough to see us in the full or even half Monty. Just as important, though, our emotions also go through adjustments in midlife, often dramatically; our spiritual needs often shift significantly as well, and our social and employment status also may alter.

If, then, we take a broader perspective consistent with the more realistic and less restrictive worldview most of us have probably developed by middle age (after all, isn't it time we admitted that photo radar will really catch only the bad drivers, that concrete is much prettier than unmowed brown grass, that not everyone on welfare is desperate to get a job, and that Microsoft is not really out to own everything—actually, scratch that last one), we can also learn to accept a much wider definition of menopause that applies to men as well. A very good example of such a definition can be found in Jed Diamond's book, *Male Menopause*. "*Male menopause*," writes Diamond, "begins with hormonal, physiological, and chemical changes that occur in all men between the ages of forty and fifty-five.... These changes affect all aspects of a man's life. Male menopause is, thus, a physical condition with psychological, interpersonal, social, and spiritual dimensions."

I agree with Diamond. I believe the term "menopause," whether we apply it to men or to women, should not be restricted to hormonal changes only but rather should signify a universal passage during midlife that encompasses hormonal, physiological, biochemical, psychological, and spiritual changes that are linked to corresponding alterations in health, outlook, expectations, self-perception, relationships, family ties, and social status. Although much more Histerian—that is, long-winded, complex, and easily forgotten—this latter definition is a great deal more consistent with what we now know happens during midlife to all men and women.

But taking into account our knowledge of hormones today (and there is no doubt that we shall find new hormones in the future), we can also conclude that what happens to most middle-aged men is not nearly as hormonally driven or as dramatic as the passage that middle-aged women go through or that the common use of the term "menopause" implies. That is why many experts now prefer to call this change of life in men andropause or viropause rather than male menopause.

Indeed, it can easily be argued that for most males, adolescence (and perhaps old age too) is a much more turbulent, hormonally driven period than is midlife. Midlife is not a time of major hormonal upheaval in men. Instead, midlife men, I submit, are generally happy souls, busily navigating, to the best of our often amateurish and certainly friable abilities, an occasionally uneven continuum from early adulthood to slipperhood. We usually manage to sail through this passage, getting bruised a bit on the way but surviving largely intact, full sails up. It often takes midlife man longer to get his sails up than it used to, and sometimes he can't even get them up at all or at best only to quarter-mast, but he knows that if he just waits a day or two or sometimes seven—or if he just takes a Viagra pill—the wind is likely to return, and then it's full mast again, for one sailing at least.

Our Need to Medicalize

If there is little proof that midlife men undergo a dramatic hormonal change, why, you may wonder, is there so much interest in establishing or manufacturing a hormonally based "male menopause"? That one is easy. It's because of Western medicine's push to medicalize everything to do with health and well-being, because the more aspects of our lives that doctors and other health professionals can claim is a deviation from some norm, the more they can treat (some might say interfere with or control). And besides, coming up with new syndromes and conditions gives much work to many people who might otherwise be greeting shoppers at Wal-Mart. What's worse is that some of these self-appointed buttinskies don't seem to care at all that there is still very little agreement even among the experts about what constitutes a normal level of so many behaviours, whims, conditions, choices, habits, vapours, actions, hormones, cell counts, and even symptoms. They are still prepared to rush in with treatment if they think someone or something is not "normal."

Sometimes, however, the associations doctors make between their observations and their calculations are tenuous at best, and dangerous and misleading at worst, as is evident from an old favourite joke of mine. A scientist captures a frog. He tells the frog to jump, and the frog leaps four feet. He then cuts off one of the frog's legs and again tells the frog to jump. The frog now jumps three feet. The scientist then cuts off another leg and so on until the frog has no legs. "Jump," says the august investigator. The frog doesn't move. Again the scientist says, "Jump." The frog doesn't move. The scientist then publishes his study in a much respected journal with the conclusion that frogs with no legs are deaf. Sadly, there seem to be lots of deaf frogs out there.

Perhaps the most dramatic recent example is the well-known phenomenon in which so many exuberant and highly energetic kids, especially boys, are now diagnosed with Attention Deficit Hyperactivity Disorder and are put on years' worth of medications, some even for life, although often such a diagnosis is based on very questionable criteria. Many boys are being treated for just being boys.

It's no wonder, then, that not long ago the Western medical community turned so many of its huge guns on menopause, a life passage that in most other cultures is considered a normal physiological event best left to nature, the counsel of wise women who have been there and done that, and the occasional herbal remedy. Now a huge army of doctors and other self-styled experts urge over half the world's population to consider this inevitable passage a diseased state of hormone deficiency requiring urgent therapeutic intervention, not only for a few years but for the rest of their lives.

So it is that with the example of ecstatic estrogen eaters to draw on, ever growing battalions of hormone researchers have tried to find similar hormonally driven changes in men. And to no one's real surprise, they have. Thus, some andrologists have now discovered a small but growing vocal community of middle-aged men whose many symptoms improve dramatically when they are placed on hormone-replacement therapy, specifically, testosterone. The leap some of these experts have made is to conclude that most aging men should be taking hormone-replacement therapy for the last few decades of their lives.

To be sure, research reveals that most men do suffer a plethora of vague complaints as we go through middle age. You don't have to be a research genius to know that at fifty we are all much more tired than we were at twenty (I'm even more tired this week than I was last week), that all of our energies—sexual, emotional, physical, social—are not what they were when we were young bucks, that we don't heal as quickly as we used to, that we are more disabled by colds and flus and other transitory conditions than we once were (at least we complain more), that it often takes us longer to get going in the morning and longer to get to sleep, that our memories and ability to concentrate may not be what they once were. But except for a very small minority of men who suffer a sharp, measurable drop in hormone levels with age, in most men, there is no proof that these symptoms are associated with a fall in their hormone levels.

MIDLIFE CRISIS—IS A CHANGE OF WIFE INEVITABLE?

But what about those notorious men who do flip out in middle age, the guys who are said to suffer "midlife crisis," a supposed hormonal hurricane that leads directly to liposuction, a hair transplant, courses in solo sailing and paragliding, a souped-up overpriced sports car, and the overthrow of a stable, long-term marriage for a fling with Kimberly or Brittany or Chelsea, a twenty-something gum-chewing Spice Girl clone. Isn't the Hollywood-endorsed male midlife crisis a universal, hormonally based phenomenon? Aren't all marriages, formalized in religious ceremonies or not, threatened by a panicky midlife male fleeing his newly recognized coop? Certainly this is a common view. But is it the right one?

In a word, no. Not only is there no proof of a link between hormones and midlife crisis, but even more surprising, perhaps, the research indicates that very few men go through a midlife crisis. On the contrary, midlife is a balanced and even tame time for most men. One expert, Dr. Larry Bumpass, has written that "midlife is a time of relative stability in marital status as most marriages and marital disruptions precede midlife and most widowhood occurs at older ages" (and I don't know about you, but I was very happy to read that last bit about widowhood occurring later). Research from the American-based John D. and Catherine T. MacArthur Foundation Research Network on Successful Midlife Development (MIDMAC), one of the few institutions that has studied midlife adults, indicates that only about 5 per cent of men have a true midlife crisis. Other surveys have come up with slightly higher numbers, although in many cases, the experts comment, this self-diagnosed crisis actually had little to do with the changes that can be ascribed to midlife. In other words, many of those men were heading for trouble anyway and their crises just happened to coincide with midlife.

What will be even more reassuring to most wives, though, is that the men who do suffer a midlife crisis are usually not the average Joes either. Researchers describe them as guys who tend to be selfish and immature, the kind of guys who weigh everything according to how it affects them ("But enough about me. Let's talk about you now. So tell me, what do you think about me?") and who hate dealing with personal or family problems. Instead of confronting an uncomfortable interpersonal situation, especially at home, these guys prefer to run away from it (can you even imagine a male who doesn't want to deal right away with a problem his wife confronts him with?) Thus, reports Winifred Gallagher in *Atlantic Monthly*, "people [read: men] prone to mid-life crisis score low on tests of introspection, or reflecting on one's self and on life, and high in denial, or coping with trouble by not thinking about it."

I suppose it also helps if they can afford to not think about it. It's not a fluke, I think, that so many of the men who seem to suffer upheavals in midlife are men with enough money to buy themselves fancy gadgets and giggling Gidgets to try to stem the perceived ebb of their manhood. Even for those guys, though—that minority of men who do endure an obvious midlife crisis—there is no credible evidence to link this "tohu vabohu" with a hormonal surge or a hormonal brownout related to their age.

So what does happen to a man in middle age? And how do most of us handle it?

Man Looking Up

Perhaps the best way to start this discussion is with a description of the typical man's life as he stands on the verge of middle age. A man in his early or mid-thirties no longer believes he will live forever, but he has not yet acknowledged that this is really all there is either. A guy in his thirties is still under the illusion that he will eventually realize all those conquering dreams he still has, that his magnificent talents will be acknowledged one day and he will assuredly rise considerably higher in the employment pecking order, that he will be able to retire before he's an old geezer of sixty—or if not retire, he will surely be enjoying the bountiful fruits of his inevitable much higher income— that his spouse (real or still just imagined) will be the exception and that he will still be making love to her (or him) on the kitchen counter in his sixties (which, by the way, is why I never accept dinner invitations from young friends, although my wife says that's more because they never invite me; she may be right but I wouldn't go anyway), that his kids (many still sperm 'n' eggs) will unquestionably grow up to play for both the Yankees and the symphony, and that if he has the time and the will, he might one day allow his name to be entered as a candidate for head of state, or even better, for the NBA.

In short, a thirty-five-year-old man hasn't grown up yet.

That's the good part of being a thirty-something: our grandest dreams are still largely intact, even though our instincts and our spouses have begun to whisper otherwise, and by the time we hit forty, of course, for many of us, those whispers have turned into shouts. The bad news is that a man within hailing distance of forty is also often submerged under a great deal of stress on all fronts—from his job, from his creditors, from his still meagre income and savings, from his kids, from his parents and in-laws, and most, perhaps, from his own expectations.

Then comes forty. Forty hits most men like a ton of bricks because it marks a cosmetic watershed, the age when most men first notice that they really do look an awful lot like their fathers; when they first reluctantly begin to accept that the growing layer of fat around their middles will never go away and that they are doomed from then on to resemble buoys more than boys; when they realize that "the legs" just don't have it anymore and that it's time to play in the nonchecking oldtimers' league; when they become aware that, on the dance floor, they now look like those cheesy old men they had always derided for working so hard at trying to look like younger bucks; when they have to acknowledge that those bald spots on their heads are not going to grow over but may soon end up looking like helicopter landing pads; when they first realize that Time's winged chariot is closing fast (and if you are wondering why a weekly news magazine would send out chariots to pursue anyone, you really should have paid more attention in your high school English class).

Forty is when most men stop looking in mirrors and when they stop taking hits. In short, forty is when they finally start growing up.

Unfortunately, it takes many men several years to get used to the idea that they are no longer young bucks with unlimited potential. This doesn't mean that during that time they are constantly lamenting their lost youth or anxiously contemplating their mortality. It does mean, though, for many men entering their forties, that their emotional and psychological well-being becomes a bit shakier. After all, at forty, most of us are still physically healthy and most of us are probably at or near our peak earning capacity, so we should be feeling great about ourselves. But for many men, the cosmetic wallop that forty kicks us with, the chop to the head and the hit in the hamstrings, can significantly dampen the seemingly good fortune of being a forty-year-old in charge.

Man at His Peak

Once we accept that turn in our lives, however, most of us seem to come out of it feeling pretty good. In fact, fifty-year-old men are the self-assessed happiest demographic group. According to data from Statistics Canada, for example, in surveys taken in 1978 and 1991, men (and women) between forty-five and sixty-four were most likely of all the demographic groups to claim a "high level of psychological well-being." And a National Center for Health Statistics survey of 44,000 Americans found that the happiest Americans were white middle-aged males living in the suburbs.

But what is this "high level of psychological well-being"? According to the MIDMAC folks cited earlier:

> There are six components of psychological well-being. These are having a positive attitude toward oneself and one's past life (self-acceptance), having goals and objectives that give life meaning (purpose in life), being able to manage complex demands of daily life (environmental mastery), having a sense of continued development and self-realization (personal growth), possessing caring and trusting ties with others . . . and being able to follow one's own convictions.

And why are these elements of psychological health most in balance at midlife? Partly because so many of us are on mood-altering drugs. More important reasons, however, are biology and control.

If biology truly is destiny, as some would have it, then happily for a man in midlife, he no longer has to deal with the dramatic biological changes of adolescence and early adulthood, and he is not yet generally slave to his biological destiny of failing health. We midlife men may complain a lot about our bodies, and we may also have lots of symptoms (complaints and symptoms do not necessarily correspond, especially for men), but we are generally pretty healthy, and our health promises to stay stable for a while.

More important, I think, midlife man usually has as much control over the social and economic aspects of his life and over his relationships as he is ever likely to have. And control, I believe, is the key to happiness, even if your health is poor. A study from Sweden concludes that even for those in their eighties and nineties, "physical frailty can be offset by an undimmed sense of mastery" or "the feeling of being actively in charge of your own life." And if this is true for ninety-year-olds, it's also certainly true for fifty-year-olds.

The control that midlife man exerts over his life is manifested in several ways. For example, contrary to the common view that many marriages stay intact only until the kids leave home and then the male partner also departs to link up with his true soulmate—some bimbo he met recently who never heard of Hamlet but who knows everything there is to know about Oasis—if you're still married when you're fifty, research shows that your marriage has either already begun to improve or else it's likely to do so soon—so long as it's the kind of marriage that

still has room for improvement, that is. Why? Because by age fifty or
so, midlife man's partner (gay or straight) has often gone through a
transition similar to his and is just as eager to get on with the rest of
his or her life. In addition, if midlife man has had kids, they are probably now at that stage where he has packed them off (many have, of
course, stormed off or sneaked off on their own), thus reinvigorating
his relationship with his partner, and if the kids' departure doesn't
always reinvigorate the relationship, then it at least allows the couple
more time and energy to work things out. Men, after all, are notorious
for slipping off, for avoiding confrontation, for retreating when any
opportunity presents itself to march away, and most men would
prefer to let marital conflicts fester, in the hope that they (the conflicts, not the men) will wither and die. It is, however, much harder to
avoid confronting a marital problem when there are only the two of
you in the house. Thus, it's likely that in midlife most marital disputes
tend to be settled earlier and more quickly than they used to be and
without becoming as corrosive as early-marriage disagreements can
get. This state of affairs not only enhances the marriage but is also
ultimately much better for a man's health (see the section on stress in
Chapter 7).

It should be no surprise, then, that according to a study in *Social
Psychology Quarterly*, if you can hang in with the same partner for
twenty-five to thirty-five years, chances are that you and your mate will
be very happy again, perhaps even as happy as you were as newlyweds.
This study claims that following the honeymoon period in a marriage,
a length of rope the study assumes lasts about four to five years, most
relationships go through increasingly rocky times as a result of the
familial responsibilities that absorb so much of our time, energy,
spirit, and money, while also giving us so much of our satisfaction.
After twenty-five years, however, this study claims, relationships start
to improve because there are fewer parental and work responsibilities,
as well as "an increase in assets," although judging from my own situation, I'm not sure how much you can count on an increase in your
assets as you boom into your fifties. You can, however, count on the
shrinking of your responsibilities just as soon as your kids are out
the door. Even better, when the kids are finally gone, many parents
establish even stronger ties with their newly adult kids, based on
mutual respect. On the parents' side, the respect stems from the relief
that their kids turned out all right after all. On the kids' side, the

respect comes from their realization that Dad wasn't really as dumb as he seemed all those years. (I'm still waiting for my sons to tell me that, by the way, but hey, even my eldest has only been gone three years.)

In middle age we often establish better relationships with our parents as well. In our middle years we may become afraid that our parents are going to die before we make our peace with them, and our parents are usually finally willing to accept that we are not going to change much anymore. My mother, for example, has finally accepted that I am never going to become a specialist—she has taken to calling me a "personality" instead, which isn't quite as good as say an allergist or a dermatologist, but it is certainly better in the Florida Jewish women's pecking order than being "just a G.P."—and that has made a big difference in our relationship.

For some men (and I count myself among them), around fifty is when they first begin to realize that in the not-too-distant future they may become grandparents and to look forward to preventing all those imperfections that, despite their undoubted parenting skills, marred their own kids.

So most family relationships and marriages, like fine wines and cheese, smell better with age. But what about work? Surely, some of you would say, work can't possibly smell better at fifty. And indeed, it often does not. One of the most significant changes for midlife men is how we view, and are viewed in, our working lives. Most men define themselves to a great extent by the kind of achievers or providers they are. Young men are not so much what they eat as what they do, and in our formative adult years, we revel in the prospect of being the best ever at whatever we have chosen to do.

By our late forties, however, and sometimes well before that, most of us have stopped dreaming about becoming the CEO, the head announcer, the judge, the dean, the foreman, even the head con on the cell block, because by then we have grudgingly accepted that we have climbed about as high as we are going to climb in our particular job or calling or prison unit. By the age of fifty, most men are aware that even if we were to attempt to scale them, there are few occupational or vocational mountains available for us to climb, since base camps on those mountains are reserved for younger folk. Quite unexpectedly, for many men, the realization that this is just about it, that we are now nearly out from under the canopy of gradually expanding expectations, comes as a great relief and allows us to look elsewhere—to the community or to our families, for example, or even inwards—for new challenges and rewards. Thus, a recent study found that the happiest and hardest-working volunteers in community organizations were people in later midlife, and these were also the people who seemed to get the most psychological satisfaction out of volunteer work.

Also, by fifty, most men have stopped trying to compete in the game immortalized, as all great ideas are these days, in a bumper sticker that reads something like: "The guy with the most toys in the end wins." Happily, many of us have achieved a certain measure of comfort by our fifties, and we have probably bought nearly every contraption, gadget, and objet d'art that we or our partners would ever want to buy, and certainly we have most of the things we absolutely need, except, perhaps, for a leather toilet seat and a sterling silver grape slicer. This realization too provides many men with a great sense of relief. I mean, you can't begin to imagine how much less stress I've had in my life ever since my wife conceded that the last renovation we did on the kitchen was probably the last kitchen renovation I would ever have to live through. Our contractor is devastated, however.

Most men also get much comfort when they hit fifty from finally admitting to themselves and to their mates that those unrealistic dreams they postponed "for a while, you know, just so I can first get ahead with my job," will never actually be realized. This necessary insight allows us to finally stop dreaming and to concentrate on real life instead of reel life. I, for example, have now accepted that I will never learn to like herbal tea (I aimed low in some of my goals), I will never play for the Montreal Canadiens, and I will never win the Nobel Prize. Well, not for peace, anyway. Literature? That's still open, I think. The obscure Polish poet and the unpopular Italian playwright categories are already filled, but the Canadian white Jewish male (Richler, Cohen, and moi) category is not, so hey, I've got a shot.

Another benefit of becoming middle-aged is that we can finally admit that the world is not as simple and that some of the good guys are not nearly as good as we've always maintained. We can finally acknowledge that those left-wing politicians we used to support turned out to be even more arrogant and greedy and cynical than the other guys, just as our dads predicted. It's ok to admit that to ourselves now and to vote for the other guys again, although we may not want to reveal it to our friends. For most midlife men it also comes as a great relief to be able to hand over responsibility for whales, dolphins, rain forests, animal experimentation, ozone, tobacco, and so on to a younger generation, whose members don't yet have lawns, mortgages, hemorrhoids, and retirement funds to worry about.

In short, a fifty-year-old man has finally grown up, and he takes a lot of satisfaction from the successes he has achieved.

Man Looking Down

All is not always as rosy as I've painted it, of course. For some middle-aged men, taking care of our kids is replaced by having to take care of our parents. These days the media, which love to profile baby-boomer concerns, abound with stories about fifty-year-olds who have become saddled with the economic and even logistic responsibility for their aging parents and perhaps for their aging in-laws as well. The happy news is that not only do most of us handle this burden with our usual aplomb but also it is not nearly as big a problem as the media have painted it to be. Today many aged parents are still quite independent, thank God, many defiantly so. Besides, quite a few of our parents are happily very far away and all they want from us is a bit of long-distance advice, although the task of advising your seventy-plus-year-old mom who lives three thousand miles away about selling her house and her lifelong accumulation of schmattes to move into a smaller apartment or—heavens!—a seniors' complex can be quite daunting.

In addition, these days, many fifty-year-olds are worried about the effect the economy and the changing social and political climate might have on their lives, especially on their jobs, before they are ready to get out. In some industries and professions, a fifty-year-old middle-class man has become an expendable commodity. And if you haven't been a good saver, fifty can seem very close to sixty-five.

Midlife is also when most of us discover that we no longer matter as much or at all to "chicks." As a man I know who claims he has bedded many women and who still looks about ten years younger than his real age of fifty-five put it to me one day, "It's really scary, man, because the young, good-looking chicks just don't look at me any longer." Although I could understand his lament—the good-looking chicks haven't looked at me for many years, if they ever did—I could not understand his panic (or the reason he still talks like a teenager). After all, why should a young woman, who has to be careful about the quality of the DNA she accepts into that single egg she will deliver that month, want to be impregnated by an older, perhaps less healthy DNA specimen when she can have her pick of younger and more desirable DNA?

Happily, most middle-aged men accept this change in our sexual status, albeit somewhat ruefully, and we generally go gentle into the next stage of our sexual maturity. (An old joke: A man of a certain age is accosted by a younger attractive woman who whispers an offer into his ear, "Super sex." "I'll take the soup," he replies instantly.) Some middle-aged men, however, are overwhelmed by this disappearing interest from the younger members of the other side, which explains why a disproportionate number of these guys seek out a trophy wife (or if they're Hollywood stars—such as Michael Douglas, Robert Redford, Harrison Ford, or Jack Nicholson—a young chicklet to co-star with) to give the world the metaphoric finger and to let everyone know that "Hey! I'm still as desirable as I ever was. Just look at this woman on my arm. She proves that the chicks still dig me." The only problem is that this guy has to wake up every morning next to someone who, when he tells her that the day Kennedy died is still perhaps the most meaningful and formative moment in his life, can't figure out why this geezer next to her would get so worked up about that guy who ran into a tree while skiing.

Of far more concern to most men is that around fifty is when most of us feel the first intimations of our mortality. This is generally when we first start to worry about getting sick, or worse, dying, and not having purchased enough life insurance. This is usually hammered home to us by news of someone our age who is either very sick or who may even have died. "Did you hear about Brian? Keeled over. Right in the middle of the deli. I never trusted those pickles, you know. What do you mean his doctor said the pickles had nothing to do with it? What do those doctors know anyway?" So for some men, fifty is also the age of panic, when men determine to do all those healthy lifestyle things they should have been doing all along.

And then there are the guys who probably take the arrival of midlife the hardest, those middle-aged men who have attained a great deal of power—and after all, despite their bleating, middle-aged guys (especially those of no colour) are still by and large the ones who run the world. Such men tend to see midlife changes as a real threat not only to their power but to their entire sense of self. To these guys, the physical changes of midlife—the belly, the wrinkles, the thinning hair, the fatigue—represent weakness, vulnerability, the passing of their king-of-the-hill potency, blood to the hordes of younger people baying at their heels. To a large extent, these are the guys who flock to doctors desperate to find a solution, preferably a hormonal or chemical one, to temporarily derail the inevitable by reversing any signs of aging and by allaying any symptoms they have, especially those symptoms that stand as public indications of their declining youthful vigour (some symptoms don't stand of course; in fact, the problem is just the opposite). These are the men so desperate to stay young and powerful forever that they will do anything, believe anything, that tells them they are not as old as the calendar says they are.

The Way It Is

So that's how guys are at middle age. Some are threatened, a few are devastated, most are happy and satisfied—at least as happy as they are ever going to be. That is why I take issue with those New Age authors and gurus who are trying to convince middle-aged guys that they are not really as happy as they think, that they need more purpose in life, and that they should be busily preparing for the next phase, in which they will become mentors and purveyors of wisdom to the younger men following behind them. Well, I've got news for those self-appointed experts: that message is, to once again quote my sagacious son, "a load of crap." First, we're not unhappy. Most of us are doing all right, Jack. Second, we're still busy; got no time to mentor. Most important, though, the men behind us are no dummies, and even if they were, that would make them no different from what we were like at their age. The guys coming up behind us don't want to hear from us, just as I never wanted to hear my father's advice until it was too late to benefit from it. I used to cringe and even leave the room when my dad used the word "experience" when he was trying to teach me something, mostly because I never wanted to experience what he had endured ("Experience," said Oscar Wilde, "is the name every one gives to their mistakes"), and with typical youthful arrogance I was equally certain that he had never experienced what I was going through. Things are no different today, of course. In what I can only think of as appropriate retribution for what I did to my dad, my sons now cringe whenever I insert that terrifying phrase "when I was your age . . ." into anything I tell them. Rather than leave the room, they begin to laugh, at which point I leave the room.

So despite the wailing of the men-who-drum and their leaders, the truth is that no matter how prepared we are to give it, the men and boys behind us don't want our insight, our accumulated wisdom, the knowledge we have gleaned from hard experience. They just want us outta here ASAP so that they can take over sooner.

And so it should be. Middle age is not a preparatory stage for mentoring but should be enjoyed for itself. What we must do is revel in our moment as the happiest demographic group around and from this self-satisfied perch build on what we have so that we are better able to handle the inevitable trials of old age. For now, while you're still in the bloom of middle age, you're "king of the world" (although I sincerely hope that if you turn your attention to writing, you produce better stuff than the drivel in *Titanic*), and it's time to enjoy being king.

I'll close this section by quoting the words of Ronald Kessler, a sociologist at MIDMAC (cited by Winifred Gallagher in *Atlantic Monthly*), who has said, "the data show that middle age is the very best time in life." In fact, "the best year is fifty." Why? Because, says Kessler, "you don't have to deal with the aches and pains of old age or the anxieties of youth. . . . You're healthy. You're productive. You have enough money to do some of the things you like to do. You've come to terms with your relationships, and the chance of divorce is very low. Midlife is the 'it' you've been working toward."

CHAPTER 2

Why Do I Look and Feel the Way I Do?

It's not the men in my life, it's the life in my men.

—MAE WEST, *I'm No Angel*

So believe it or not, fifty is the "it" you have relentlessly been marching towards all those formative years. That's the good news. The inevitable bad news, however, is that "it" is not quite nirvana. Although "it" clearly beats whatever lies in second place (the current only known alternative to turning fifty is not turning fifty), "it" is often accompanied by some unwelcome physical alterations.

Before I move on to discuss those changes, however, I have to offer a disclaimer. For those of you who have been lured into buying this book by reading the dust jacket, which implies that a disproportionate amount of the text is devoted to sexual matters and sexual parts, my deep apologies. To be sure, that is certainly what my publisher wanted. "Sex sells," he pointedly mentioned, even before I had written the first paragraph. Indeed, every time he called me to discuss the project, he invariably whined something like, "Couldn't you put just a bit more sex into it, Art? At the very least, can't you move the sex parts up to the front where they belong?"

There is a common misconception that if sex is not the only health issue that matters to men, young, middle-aged, and old, it is certainly the most important one, a belief seemingly borne out by the frenzy over Viagra. Now I suppose this is true for some men, but even penis-driven ever ready automatons who just keep coming and coming and coming usually realize as they begin to age that man cannot live by bed alone, which is why even most of them are just as interested in and concerned about the changes that occur to their other body parts and functions. I will concede, however, that sex is very important, and so it has been given its own chapter (Chapter 3). For now we will concentrate on all those other changes that happen to your body as you hit your middle years.

That Sagging Skin

For a startling example of the difference between your middle-aged skin and the skin of a younger person, here's an easy experiment you can try at home or in a pub. First, after obtaining permission, of course, gently pinch a younger person's skin, preferably skin in a sun-exposed area. See how quickly it snaps back into place? Now pinch your own skin and watch as it slowly sinks back to a semblance of flatness. See how long it takes? Your skin has begun to dry out; hers has not yet started to.

In middle age, skin has begun to sag and desiccate and bunch up and wrinkle and prune. It also becomes less elastic and more mottled, and you begin to notice an increasing number of those small blood vessels that are a sure giveaway of aging skin. And as we all know from the Marlboro Man, these normal components of aging may be greatly accentuated by accumulated damage from excess exposure to the sun and from smoking.

These changes can be very disturbing. A survey done for Ortho Pharmaceuticals and published in *USA Today* found that wrinkles disturb boomers more than grey hair does, probably because so many middle-aged guys don't have enough hair to be concerned about its colour, although they certainly have lots of wrinkles to worry about. To minimize these changes, stay out of the sun as much as possible. Your time as a bronzed sun god has come and most assuredly gone. Cover up. And don't smoke, of course.

As to treatment, a growing number of my peers have begun to visit plastic surgeons—excuse me, cosmetic surgeons. According to the American Academy of Cosmetic Surgery, the percentage of men consulting these snip-and-tuckers rose from 10 per cent in 1980 to 24 per cent in 1994, which I guess still leaves a whole lot of guys who should go but haven't gone yet. There is a cornucopia of choices open to you—botulism toxin injections, collagen injections, peels, nose jobs, liposuction, face-lifts, and who knows what else. If you have the money and the inclination, then by all means, rearrange.

If you're not into surgery, however, you could always mimic our sisters by using alpha-hydroxy acid creams or tretinoin, a derivative of vitamin A, to hide the effects of aging and ultraviolet radiation damage. These creams have been shown to improve wrinkling, surface roughness, and even some of the colour changes that occur in photo-damaged skin. A real man would never resort to such artifice, however, and besides, when I used it, the tretinoin was very irritating.

THE HAIR APPARENT

As we age, our hair begins to lose colour and turn grey because of a fall in the number of active melanocytes, the cells that govern skin and hair pigment. In addition, the number of hair follicles on our scalp decreases, and the rate of growth of the hair in the still active follicles also slows, often to a metaphoric crawl. I once required a haircut every three weeks; I now get my hair attended to only once every six weeks, and even then my stylist (she used to be my barber back when I used to be her doctor, not her health care provider) spends more time trimming my wallet than the back of my scalp. In God's great joke, however, while hair on our scalp becomes thinner and sparser in middle age, hair on other parts of our bodies starts to grow, even to blossom, which is why most middle-aged guys have to regularly and painfully extract hair growing out of various openings in their skulls.

Male-pattern baldness can be inherited from a male on either side of the family, and I got my dad's hair, I'm afraid, along with his great looks and sweet nature too, of course. Hair loss in young and middle-aged men is a lot more common than you may think. Twenty per cent of men start to lose hair by age twenty-five, and in a recent study, researchers concluded that by middle age, 50 per cent of men have some of what they call MPHL, which sounds more like a hockey league than what it really stands for—male-pattern hair loss. This study also found, as you would expect, that men make more of a to-do about their do than do neutral observers, because for a balding man his hair loss is an embarrassingly public signal of growing old. No surprise, then, that Americans spent an estimated $1.5 billion on balding therapies last year.

So what have I done about my hair loss, you are no doubt wondering if you have seen my picture on the dust jacket. To be honest, I twice tried to do something about it. First, as a much younger man, on the advice of my hirsute barber (I think he was a Rastafarian—he always wore one of those caps, and there was always an interesting smell in the shop; that's why I kept going back), I purchased some mustard oil and diligently applied it to my scalp for a few weeks. Although he had assured me that the mustard oil would slow down my hair loss, all that it did was make my scalp burn and make me smell terrible. For some worrisome reason, though, no one seemed to treat me any differently.

The second therapy I tried was Rogaine, or topical minoxidil, a shampoo that is now available in a couple of strengths and that does work for a small proportion of men; it did nothing for me, however. You can also try Propecia, a small dose of the prostate drug finasteride (see Chapter 4). Both Rogaine and Propecia can produce modest increases in hair growth, but you had better have deep pockets to go with your shiny scalp because the minute you discontinue these drugs, you start losing hair again. Furthermore, we still have no idea what using these drugs for many years will do to you (such as, for example, give you hairy palms from applying the shampoo regularly). Minoxidil is, after all, a blood-pressure-lowering medication that can, even in shampoo form, affect certain measures of heart function, and finasteride interferes with the conversion of testosterone to another form of the hormone. Thus, both of these drugs may still prove to have deleterious long-term effects on health. Other side effects of Propecia include loss of libido and impotence, and there is probably nothing more frustrating than to be well coifed but with no interest or ability to go where your hair is willing to take you.

After these two self-administered treatments, you are left with rugs and slugs, the former referring to hairpieces, of course, the latter being my term for the always cautious and slow cosmetic surgeons who make fortunes off the various surgical procedures required to make your scalp look like, well, a scalp that has had hair transplanted onto it.

The most exciting possibilities on the horizon are one, gene therapy, and two, estrogen blockers. The latter seem promising because of a recent finding that excess estrogen may play a key role in some cases of male-pattern baldness (although certainly not in mine), and so researchers are hot on the trail of a cream or pill that blocks the estrogen effect on the scalp.

Finally, the best thing to do may just be to grin and bare it. There is a rather pleasant compensation to baldness, you see, and that is that many people equate lack of hair on the scalp with extra brain matter in the cranium. According to a study from Denison University in Ohio, both men and women claimed that bald men in the pictures they looked at were smarter than their more hirsute brothers. The bad news is that the balding men were also judged to be much less attractive—but that's not as bad as it seems because you can always get some plastic surgery, but you can't get a transplant of grey matter.

Getting Fatter While Your Bones Get Thinner

Perhaps the most depressing study I came across in my research is one that concluded that unless a middle-aged man continually increases the number of calories he burns every day, he will inevitably get fatter, a finding easily verified by perusing any typical sports arena, where so many middle-aged guys look as if they're training to become Michelin Man stand-ins. Middle-aged men also begin to lose muscle mass (yes, I had to assure my wife, even men who have no discernible muscles to begin with) as our muscle tissue starts to weaken and shrink. As well, our bones begin to thin slowly from middle age on. Although degenerative arthritis is still not common in midlife, middle-aged men begin to complain of more aches and pains than they did when younger, and they find that it takes longer to recover from nagging soft tissue injuries such as muscle pulls. This is all probably a reflection of increasingly inelastic ligaments and tendons, as well as less springy articular cartilage, the tissues that provide cushioning in the joints.

Exercise and a healthy diet (discussed in Chapters 6 and 7) can, of course, slow down these tendencies, although they are inevitable.

Losing Your Senses

The lens of the eye starts to thicken in middle age, leading to poorer night vision and focus, especially for close objects. That explains why many middle-agers need to work so hard to find the best distance to hold a page from our noses.

What happens to our hearing faculties as we age is best illustrated in this old story in which a middle-aged man tells a friend, "You know, my wife left me." "Why?" asks the friend. "Because she says I never listen to her. At least that's what I think she said."

Joking aside, in middle age, hearing diminishes more rapidly in men than in women, especially for higher tones (and especially for women's voices, I think).

It's unclear how much taste and smell we lose with advancing age. On the one hand, a report from Duke University claims that loss of taste and smell are common as we age. On the ever present other hand, a study from the Claude Pepper Center for Research on Oral Health at the University of Florida found that in some people the senses of touch, taste, and smell deteriorate only slightly with age—if they don't smoke or drink too much.

LUNGS AND HEART

The respiratory system becomes less efficient in middle age because the lungs start to lose some of their essential elasticity. This results in poorer oxygenation of the blood. If you're still stupid enough to smoke, middle age is when you generally begin to notice the first signs of chronic bronchitis or emphysema—chronic, persistent cough and increasing shortness of breath—and middle age is certainly when you will first begin to fear that you have lung cancer, a fear that, like *MASH* reruns and Jack Lemmon–Walter Matthau movies, will return to haunt you with increasing and sickening regularity.

In middle age, our hearts become less efficient. For many of us, our heart rate can't go up as rapidly during exercise, and our aerobic capacity also begins to fall. As well, our arteries start becoming less elastic, and the one-way valves in our veins stop being as efficient as they once were, which is why so many of us start developing varicose veins.

As usual, exercise (Chapter 7) is the key to minimizing the effects from these changes.

KIDNEYS AND BLADDER

The kidneys shrink as we get older, and their filtering efficiency also begins to fall. For me, one of the worst things about middle age is that not only does the bladder begin to have less capacity to store urine, but it also doesn't empty itself as well when you tell it to unload, which is why, dear readers, for me there is a one-minute gap in every movie I have recently seen. And when my prostate is unruly, a three-minute gap.

Falling Energy and Falling Asleep

In middle age, our energy levels fall to varying degrees, depending on the man. Some guys complain that they just don't have enough energy to get around or do some of the things they used to do as vim-filled young bucks—housekeeping duties usually but sometimes bear hunting too—while other guys don't complain at all. They just go to bed at 9:00 P.M., two hours after their wives hit the sack. No matter how we handle it, this energy drop is unavoidable, as anyone who has ever been stuck in a room full of middle-aged yawners at 9:00 P.M. can attest.

Middle-agers also sleep differently than when we were younger. Not only do we go to bed sooner, but we sleep less deeply than we used to. And according to a British study in *Occupational and Environmental Medicine*, people over the age of forty-seven also tend to rise earlier, and we tend to fade sooner than we used to after lunch; I often fade before lunch.

There are a host of strategies to help you sleep better. You can start with keeping to a regular sleep schedule. Getting married also helps, since married people tend to sleep better (and the longer you are married, the more sleep you get; see Chapter 3 on monogamy and sexual frequency). Getting rid of anything in the bedroom that might disturb your sleep, such as a TV or a flea-bitten early-rising mutt, not eating too heavily before bedtime, and getting more exercise, which has been shown in several studies to improve quality of sleep and ability to fall asleep, are sound sleep-stimulating strategies as well. You should also avoid any substance that can interfere with sleep, such as alcohol, coffee, and the many drugs that contain caffeine. And you can try a warm bath, siestas, relaxation techniques, sex (but only if it relaxes you), and a glass of warm milk or (if you can stomach such mellow stuff) camomile tea. Used cautiously, herbal sleep remedies, valerian, and melatonin can also prove useful. Melatonin, however, is not available in Canada, where the ever vigilant health police prefer to spend their time busting melatonin pushers rather than trying to get Canadians and Canadian doctors to use far less of the much more dangerous and ubiquitous medications we use so freely.

Then there's this strategy. According to advice from Professor Jim Horne of Loughborough University of Technology in the U.K. and reported in the London *Times*, warming the brain by increasing its visual workload in the daytime helps people sleep better. In other words, anything that makes the visual part of your brain work more, such as window shopping, Horne suggests, will help you sleep. Before you dismiss this suggestion as nonsense, let me tell you that I know at least one woman for whom this strategy works well, so well that she doesn't stop at the window, she actually shops to help her sleep, and believe me, she always sleeps better than I do that night. Horne says that his theory that warming the brain helps you sleep better may also explain why sitting in a nice, hot bath is such an effective sleep remedy, especially, I suppose, in those people whose brain is situated where they sit.

The Brain—How to Hang On to What's Left

A study from the University of Pennsylvania has shown that although men start out with more brain cells than women (young men need those big brains or else how could they remember all those vital sports statistics?), men also lose brain cells three times as fast as women as they age. Thus, by age forty-five, men's brains and women's brains are roughly the same size, although egos continue to remain much larger in men. This assertion that egos are larger in men has recently been supported by a study that found that although men are much more confident than women that they can remember where they left the car keys, women are actually much better than men at knowing where such misplaced items might be found—all except for the beer and nachos, I'll bet.

The loss of brain cells with age is most acute in the frontal lobes, those areas that govern cognitive functions, such as mental flexibility and attention span, a finding that might explain aging men's obsession with channel surfing and our inability to tell our wives anything important that they think we should have overheard at a cocktail party. Brain cells are also lost in the hippocampus and midbrain, and this diminution of brain matter seems to affect memory and the sense of time elapsed from a given moment. Thus, time really does seem to be catching up to you much more quickly the older you get.

But why, you may well wonder as you are busily flipping channels and not finding anything that can keep your attention for more than a millisecond, do men lose more brain cells than women do? My wife's theory is that God figured that men wouldn't miss their brain cells as much as women would, but there's no real proof of that. According to a more objective theory, we men are just not able to switch off our brains, while women can easily put their brains into neutral, an observation that any man who has ever listened to a group of women chatting will no doubt instantly affirm. Men, however, may just not be able to let go of thinking furiously about something, anything, even while at rest, not really surprising when you consider all the important things that are constantly on our minds—how to get out of doing any more work on the clunker in the garage, whether our team can beat the points spread, whether to put mustard on before the ketchup, and so on. Consequently, this theory claims, men suffer the equivalent of an overuse injury of the brain; they may "burn out" some parts of their brains more quickly than women.

Is there anything you can do to stem the ebbing tide of your cognitive functions, short of carrying around a twenty-four-page and rapidly growing list of "to do" items and wearing an "If found, please return to . . ." sign around your neck? To a certain extent, yes.

- For a start, you can stay healthy. A study from Scotland found that Scots who remain healthy into old age also maintain their full youthful intellectual abilities, although I leave it to your imagination as to how they were able to determine the difference between a Scot with diminished intellectual functions and a "normal" one. Did the researchers give them some haggis and see what they did with it? What would the right answer be anyway?
- Then you can work on your female side, since women are better than men at remembering lists and people's names.
- You should also get a good education because the higher your level of education, the better your memory in old age.
- Keep your stress level down because recent studies suggest that chronic stress leads to memory impairment.
- Keep your blood pressure down because high diastolic blood pressure in middle age has been linked to impaired cognitive abilities in later life.
- Do lots of exercise. Several excellent studies show that regular exercise retards memory loss.

You might also try to prevent brain burnout. Specifically, Dr. Ruben Gur, professor of psychiatry at the University of Pennsylvania and a leading expert in this area, told the London *Times* that "men may need to relax their brain in the same way they relax their muscles," not as much of a leap as you may think for the many men whose brains are largely muscle tissue anyway.

But relaxing your brain does not mean not using it at all. What you want to aim for is to use different parts of your brain, to exercise different brain functions than you usually do because the more flexible your brain is, the more varied stimulation it receives, the more synapses you build up over the years and the less it seems to fade with time.

And this advice is true throughout life. Thus, a study of Swedish twins concluded that 38 per cent of our ability to acquire and process knowledge is a product of our environment, and that even older adults can still process new information and learn new skills. By the way, this figure also means, unfortunately, that 62 per cent (100 less 38 equals 62, except if you're my ex-accountant, although maybe even he would come up with this answer now that he has been able to do some remedial math in prison) of our general cognitive skills in old age is a result of our genes, and that is something we can't affect.

"Absolutely terrible news," screamed my son Tim when I gave him this information. "Don't be silly," I shot back with a snide look at my wife. "You're ok. After all, you got half your brains from me." "That's what he meant," she smirked.

As to more active treatment, it is likely we will soon have drugs to rejig the brain and its functions. Although scientists have always believed that after a brain cell dies it stays dead and can never be replaced, recent research has shown that the brain can regrow some cells. Thus, it is possible that one day scientists might find a drug that can regrow some of those passed-away neurons. As well, the *New Scientist* reports that a "memory pill" is nearly here. There will be some major problems with this breakthrough drug, however—not only are you going to have to remember to take it in the first place, but you will also have to remember where you last left the pillbox.

IF THAT'S LIFE, DO I EVER NEED HELP

So there you have it—most of the changes that will happen to you as you proceed through your midlife passage. You can, however, decrease the inevitable toll that time exacts by adopting some good lifestyle habits, as described in Chapters 6 and 7. Not only are these habits the key to preventing many of the diseases and health problems you run into as you get older, but they can also slow down many of the normal aging effects you have just read about.

And what are those habits? The usual suspects:

- Don't smoke.
- Use only minimal to moderate amounts of alcohol.
- Follow a healthy diet.
- Get lots of sleep.
- Minimize your stress load.
- Probably most important, get lots of exercise.

If you don't start on that path of righteousness, brothers—and as a realist, I know that most of you heathens won't—there are really only two other ways to deal with the inevitable deterioration of age. As I have already mentioned, if you have the money and if it fits your political views, you can take the Dick Clark route—that is, get yourself a ton of plastic surgery. Although you won't reverse the deterioration in the really important bodily functions, at the very least as you get older and older, you will continue to amaze people with your skin's ability to stretch without beginning to leak. Or you can choose what is still the most popular route—just accept what the calendar throws at you and take your chances with that. If you do that, however, let me offer my condolences to your partner, mostly because he or she is the one who will have to watch you get undressed every night.

CHAPTER 3

Sex and the Middle-Aged Male

The emphasis on performance is the
single greatest enemy of a satisfactory sexual life.

—GAIL SHEEHY, "The Unspeakable Passage," *Vanity Fair*

Leonard Cohen, a man who's clearly been there and certainly done that (when I come back, I hope it's as a sour, lined, black-garbed poet), has complained in song that he aches in places where he used to play. Although most of us have not been fortunate enough to play nearly as often as Leonard has and certainly not on the same squad that Leonard managed to be drafted for, the reality is that even if we never quite made it onto the first-string team, most middle-aged guys are "aching" in places that once used to be ache-free.

Now before you leap to a fallacious conclusion, let me quickly interpose that I'm absolutely certain that Leonard is using "ache" in a metaphorical sense. It's not so much that middle-aged guys experience physical pain in the old playground; it's more that our seesaw doesn't go as high as it used to when we were younger. Some guys are even finding that they cannot get their seesaw off the ground any longer, the countervailing weight, either emotional or physical, having become too heavy to be lifted without appropriate assistance. And that is why, of course, Viagra has become this era's hula hoop and pet rock.

SEXUAL CHANGES IN MIDLIFE—GOOD TO THE LAST DROOP

What does happen to sexual functioning in middle age in men? Not much, but too much. For a start, a man's testicles shrink slightly as he

ages (and no, I don't know anyone who has actually had theirs measured, nor do I know of any health plan that would pay for this procedure should you choose to have it done), they don't ride as high as they
used to, the aging male's scrotum tends not to shrink as much when he
becomes aroused, and the number of testosterone-producing cells
begins to drop. There is also a smaller volume of pre-ejaculatory
secretions, sperm production and semen volume fall, and there is a
small drop-off in the percentage of mature sperm that are most cap-
able of fertilizing an anxious yet hopeful ovum. Overall, however, most
middle-aged men still produce enough sperm to be able to impregnate
a partner, if not quite on demand, then at least with effort, in time.
("With effort, in time," by the way, is the Hister family motto, at least
for the male side of the family.)

In addition, erections begin to change in midlife. Now I realize that
many of you, especially the younger men, might have trouble understanding that last bit. For most younger guys, after all, an erection is
much like an elevator in a three-storey tenement building—it goes up
and it goes down, the view while it's in use is generally nonvarying, and
aside from the speed at which your elevator delivers you from the
depths of the basement to the exhilaration of the penthouse, there
really isn't much else to appreciate or criticize about it. And usually,
that's the way it goes in the early years. Up and down, up and down, on
command, when in demand, zipping rapidly between floors, deliver-
ing its soon-to-be-ecstatic cargo to the luxurious upstairs suites
whenever called on to carry the weight, and requiring minimal maintenance, not even any regular lubrication for that matter. But even the
most pampered and well-maintained elevator can sometimes get stuck
between floors. It might even malfunction on occasion by lingering on
the lower-level floors. Worst of all, like HAL, the computer in *2001—A
Space Odyssey*, the elevator might even develop a mind of its own and
prefer to stay grounded most of the time, despite its handler's best
attempts to get it moving upward into service. That's how it is with
erections too, so during middle age, not only do many men begin to
suffer from occasional bouts of impotence but even a midlife man who
is always able (with effort, in time) to get hard enough to do his duty
tends to suffer a bit of loss of upward mobility of his penis due to
changes in the blood vessels that are responsible for creating and
maintaining an erection. These changes also lead to a slight alteration
in the angle of the erection.

Middle age also brings changes to the "quality" of an erection. Not only does it take most middle-aged guys longer to achieve even a garden-variety, run-of-the-mill erection, but in contrast to when they were young, when a rock-hard erection immediately sprang up after even the vaguest erotic thought, in midlife some men may require direct physical stimulation to get an erection, or they may not hit full hardness until they are in place, because erections tend to become less firm (much like other body parts of the middle-aged owner of those erections), the kind of erections that men often describe as "softer" or "weaker." How do we know that, you ask. Because the people who study these things actually have a way of measuring the strength of erections. (Those of you reading this chapter to your kids as a bedtime story might want to skip the next part.) In *Clock of Ages*, Dr. John Medina claims that "ejaculatory distance" drops off from "two feet in young men to only minimal dribbling distance in the elderly," and I'll bet you that until you read that, you had absolutely no idea that they even held that kind of competition. Well, they clearly do, and I'll bet that it's a sellout every time.

For some middle-aged men, even with physical stimulation—to paraphrase Gertrude Stein's comment about Oakland—there is often no there, there. In other words, middle age is when increasing numbers of men begin to be visited by that unwelcome guest known as impotence (see the next section), who is inevitably greeted like a death figure in a Woody Allen film, come to call on the wrong guy at the wrong time. For men who begin to be troubled by intermittent but increasingly frequent visits from this frightening apparition, a diamond-hard erection becomes elusive, and for a small but growing number of men, it becomes rarer to experience a trouble-free sexual episode than to discover a television talk show host with at least a double-digit IQ.

Midlife man also finds that his orgasm is often shorter. "But how much shorter can it get?" asked my smirking wife, proving how little attention she actually pays to what I tell her. It's orgasm that they're talking about, not foreplay. With increasing age, a man's erection also detumesces faster—that is, his rocket plummets to earth more quickly than it did in the old days, and he can't relaunch nearly as rapidly for a second flight.

These generally gradual changes are universal with advancing years, and no man is immune, but clearly they don't affect all men equally. Furthermore, no matter how mild or severe the changes may be, men respond to them in very different ways. After all, the brain, which usually includes the mind, is still the biggest and certainly the most important sexual organ for men. Thus, some guys are devastated by even the slightest change in their sexual apparatus or functioning, while others seem to absorb significant changes with only minimal complaints. Now that Viagra is available, however, even these guys are appearing in doctors' offices in amazing numbers to get help stiffening their resolve.

ARISE, YOU PRISONERS OF DEFLATION

Impotence—or as the experts now refer to it, erectile dysfunction, a name I simply loathe because it reminds me of my kids' toy erector set and how my own constructions always kept falling over ("Maybe it's a lesson for later life," my wise wife used to say)—is the inability to obtain and sustain an erection for satisfactory intercourse. Impotence is a major concern for many—actually all—men. A recent American survey found that if given the choice, men would rather go deaf and blind and end up in severe pain than have their willie wilt—that is, a majority of men said they would rather have a hearing impairment, cataracts, high blood pressure, or arthritis than impotence, although the great joke on these guys is that as typical North American men, they are likely to end up with all of the above, including impotence, anyway.

The incidence of impotence rises with age. By age forty, 5 per cent of men are frequently unable to perform when called on, while one-third of men report occasional difficulties performing. By age fifty, the "occasional" group has risen (or not) to 50 per cent of all men, and 10 to 15 per cent of fifty-year-old men are completely impotent. These numbers march steadily upwards until age seventy, when over half the male population is unable to stand at attention on demand, or even when not in demand, just hopeful. On the bright side, the Massachusetts Male Aging Study found that 40 per cent of men were still completely potent at age seventy.

In older men, everyone agrees that impotence is largely a physical problem, mostly caused by damage to the arteries that feed the penis. It's not surprising, then, that erectile difficulties are a lot more common in men whose arteries are under attack from diseases such as diabetes, coronary heart disease, and high blood pressure, as well as in men who smoke or drink heavily. Any man who begins to suffer increasing bouts of impotence should consult his doctor about the state of his arteries because impotence can be a marker for cardiovascular disease that has not shown up with other symptoms. Various metabolic, urologic, and neurologic conditions can also produce impotence, and men dealing with chronic health problems are also more prone to impotence, both from the psychological burden and from the physical toll that chronic illness exacts. In addition, many medications can affect a man's ability to perform. Finally, that small proportion of men with very low testosterone levels also suffers from impotence, although there is no connection in most men between their testosterone levels and their potency.

In younger men, the situation is a bit different. Even in middle-aged men the cause of most impotence is physical, but psychological factors probably play a larger role for that age group than for older men. For example, the Massachusetts Male Aging Study found a link between impotence and depression and repressed anger. Increased stress can also lead to impotence. Israeli researcher Dr. Alexander Oshanyesky has found that when the stock market plummets, so do men's erections, probably because, he told the London *Times*, "stress causes the adrenalin level to shoot up, moving more blood to the brain and the heart and less to the penis." This finding, by the way, also gives the lie to the claim by so many women that a man's heart never has any connection to his penis. According to Oshanyesky, there have only been two occasions in which an effective drug for impotence (which I presume is Viagra) did not have the desired effect on the men in his Israeli clinic: when Scud missiles hit Israel during the Gulf War, and during the Tel Aviv stock market crash of 1993. What I want to know, though, is what kind of man seeks out this kind of medication when Scud missiles are raining down on his country?

As to treatment, as always, an ounce of prevention is worth a pound of loin, and to that end, all the usual lifestyle prohibitions apply. Hard as it may be, don't smoke, don't drink too much, don't become fat and sedentary, and try to relax, especially in bed. After all, if you're fat and smoke a ton and drink excessively and you're always tense, you may never get a chance to find out if you even have an erectile problem in the first place. Also, if you are one of those immature guys who are still using recreational drugs at age fifty, not only do you seriously need a life, man, but until you get one, remember that overuse of all recreational drugs is linked to erectile problems.

In addition, be wary of any nonrecreational drugs you are taking. Among the many drugs that can either produce or worsen an already existing softness around the edge, the antihypertensives are especially likely to produce this effect, although digoxin, nonsteroidal anti-inflammatories, antihistamines, tranquillizers, antidepressants, and a host of others can also cause or worsen erectile difficulties. A warning, though: if you suspect that a drug you are on is leaving you limp, don't just stop it abruptly. Talk to your doctor first about perhaps switching to something that might affect you less.

As for most organs, a "use it or lose it" policy is best for the penis too. It's just like riding a bike. Even if you never quite forget how to do it, it's a lot easier to maintain your expertise, especially in traffic, than to go back and do it after a prolonged period of abstinence. Happily, this is the kind of homework most men don't resent doing.

You should also work on stress relief, but remember that impotence is not the kind of problem that you can will away. In fact, the more you focus on your inability to perform when Chip is down, the more likely you will be unable to rise the next time out. And remember that in many instances, sexual difficulties, including impotence, stem from, and are always worsened by, communication problems in a relationship. If you have such problems, consider consulting a professional therapist who is willing to see both you and your patient mate to help you sort things out.

For more active treatment, every culture has its witch doctors who promote some sort of aphrodisiac for its underachievers. I don't know what kind of a man would try some of these, but among the many products I have heard about are ginseng, deer antler extract, tiger penises, avocados, rhinoceros horns, carrots, oysters, pomegranates, honey, royal jelly, fertilized duck eggs, lobsters, caviar, prairie oysters or bulls' and rams' testicles (I found those a bit chewy, by the way), bear meat and bear gallbladder (ditto!), wild yams, licorice, and freeze-dried chicken extract.

In North America, witch doctors prefer to start with some kind of drug, preferably a prescription medication, and to that end, the drug sildenafil (Viagra) has recently been introduced to great acclaim in the United States. Viagra works by blocking an enzyme that allows blood to flow out of the penis. Thus, with Viagra, the penis engorges and stays filled until it's done its duty. Viagra is said to be successful in up to 80 per cent of men with either physically based or psychologically based impotence when taken as a pill one hour before it is needed. In the prerelease studies, some men who took Viagra were able to become erect three times a night, causing some experts to worry about the "potential for abuse" or "addiction." This is abuse? Certainly not where I come from.

And clearly, millions of men around the world agree with me. Pfizer Inc., the makers of Viagra, reported that pharmacists in the United States filled more than six hundred thousand prescriptions for Viagra the first month it was available, and a hot market in Viagra sales has sprung up overseas as well. I'm sure that even the Messiah would have trouble getting that many men to stand at attention for him. In fact, Pfizer Inc. was so enthusiastic about Viagra sales that the company has begun immediate and intensive research to find the next Holy Grail of science, a faster-acting Viagra.

So why shouldn't we all run out and get ourselves some Viagra? For a start, most of us don't need it. In theory, Viagra does not enhance normal erections, although the jury is still out on that one (and the jury members are probably experimenting with Viagra on their own to find out). Viagra is not an aphrodisiac and doesn't work in the absence of sexual stimulation. Viagra also doesn't work in every man. In addition, I hate to be the one who sees a naked emperor, but at least some of Viagra's oomph is due to a placebo effect (in the studies, at least one-quarter of men responded equally well to a placebo), and for men who are being pumped up by false pretenses, prairie oysters are a whole lot cheaper, though they may be harder to obtain. Viagra also produces side effects, such as (and women all over the world are laughing at this) precoital headaches, flushing, nasal stuffiness, and abdominal discomfort.

More seriously, a small but significant proportion of men who take Viagra, especially those taking higher doses, experience a change in their perception of colour and brightness, and they develop a "bluish" vision. The long-term consequences of these visual changes are clearly not established. It's possible that in some men—such as diabetic men, who are at higher risk for both blindness and impotence (see Chapter 5)—this kind of love really might leave them blind. Most seriously, though, Viagra also lowers blood pressure, especially in men who are taking nitroglycerin or other nitrates for angina (chest pain as a result of activity). Thus, men on nitrates should avoid Viagra.

My main beef with this baby-boomer sexual aid, however, is that

Viagra does only one thing for its user. It gets the machine ready to work. But sexual performance is not the same as sexual intimacy, and the male obsession with performance to the exclusion of the rest of what is essential for a vital and healthy sexual relationship will, I believe, lead to trouble in many relationships. The ram in the bedroom may not be as welcome to the ewe as he thinks. In a great column for the *New York Times*, Maureen Dowd claimed that "what's wrong with these would-be-studs [who bought Viagra in the first week it was out] pills can't fix." She went on. "An unscientific poll of my girl-friends found that they would rather have a pill that could change a man's personality an hour *after* sex. A pill that insures that he always calls the next day and never gets spooked." Most women would probably agree with that.

For those who can't or won't take Viagra, you can try the drug yohimbine, although it probably helps only a small minority of men. Other oral therapies include phentalomine and zinc. Oral alprostadil is used in some countries, but postmarketing studies are still not available, so buyer beware. Testosterone-replacement therapy usually doesn't help much with impotence (except in men with very low testosterone levels), although testosterone replacement does increase the urge to try to venture where you know you will only tread softly.

A medication that received a standing ovation in a report from England was nitroglycerin, either in a paste or patch form. According to this study, four of ten men got an erection within two hours of applying the patch and were able to maintain the erection for up to three hours, time enough to smuggle the goods a pretty fair distance. The only significant side effects were headaches and an unfortunate tendency to explode if the subjects wandered too close to a match.

Pellets of alprostadil that are pushed three centimetres into the urethra have recently been introduced in some markets—gently, I hope. In many men, however, these pellets may not produce the quality of erection required to make an impotent man happy. In addition, questions remain about the long-term safety of this therapy.

Until Viagra rocketed in, the mainstay of impotence therapy was some kind of mechanical solution—vacuum suction cylinders, surgically implanted penile inflatable prostheses, and injections. The use of these therapies has plummeted, however, since Viagra rose to grab the market.

Finally, a word about something you should not do to try to improve your sexual performance. According to a survey from McGill University, reported in the *Medical Post*, "a bigger penis does not cure impotence." (It's great to see, by the way, that my alma mater is still on the cutting edge of science.) But what the hell does that mean, you are no doubt wondering. Not what you think. What it means is that cosmetic surgery to enlarge the penis as well as techniques in which the veins to the penis are tied off in an attempt to get blood to stay in the penis longer do not correct erectile or sexual problems. In fact, if you do have what you consider to be a small penis, take heart in a couple of observations. First, when erect, even most smaller penises are big enough to do whatever jobs they are given. Second, a recent theory has proposed that body parts may compete for size during development, so the good news is that your smaller penis may simply be a reflection of your larger brain. Or maybe just your larger spleen. Whatever.

RATES OF SEXUAL INTERCOURSE—LIAR, LIAR

The common belief is that frequency of sexual intercourse slips, generally bit by bit, but occasionally much more dramatically, as we age, a belief that is borne out in most surveys (although Viagra may eventually change that). But before you get too melancholy about a middle life and old age restricted to checkers and shuffleboard, bear in mind that in surveys about sex, there is always another hand. So on the other hand, I have seen at least two hopeful surveys. One found that 30 per cent of men over the age of eighty claimed they were still having intercourse at least once a week, while the other found that one in five Canadian men over the age of seventy says he's still having sex weekly. That's weekly, and not weakly, by the way, although it's often both, of course.

I must warn you, however, that I would take this latter survey with a grain of salt because it also found that only one in fifteen Canadian women over age seventy said that they have sex weekly. So how can we explain this discrepancy between the Canuck old guys and gals? The possibilities are that one in five elderly Canadian men is a liar (impossible!), that those geezers are bedding younger women in droves (also hard to believe if you live in Canada and get a chance to see our hordes of grizzled, pucklike, older gents), that they are having sex with each other (perish the thought), or that they are having lots of virtual sex and lots of sex with themselves, which makes me wonder in turn about the 80 per cent of Canadian senior men who aren't even doing that.

By the way, this kind of discrepancy is not unique to Canadian sex surveys. Similar discrepancies between what men claim and what women claim about how often they have sex have also been found in surveys from the United States, Great Britain, and Norway. Wherever you look, it seems, men think, or at least say, they have more sex than women.

But no matter what the numbers say, the important point is that sex surveys have very little relevance for thee and me because how frequently each of us has sexual intercourse depends on many factors that affect each of us differently. For a start, for most of us, sexual intercourse tends to occur much more often if we have a partner to share this experience with. As we men age, however, our ability to hang on to a partner, or to discover a new partner, willing to do it as often as we want to do it, is frequently more difficult than it was when we were younger. For most of us, it was also tough to find such a partner when we were younger, but at least the chances were better then.

A man's emotional and psychological state also affects the frequency with which he has or even wants to have intercourse. Thus, men who are depressed or under lots of stress tend to have much less intercourse than their carefree, play-it-as-it-lays brothers. Since the brain is the most important sexual organ, as we age, our sexual functioning is also affected by the variable although inevitable neurological and brain changes that occur with advancing age, including alterations in the levels of some neurotransmitters in the brain.

Other factors that affect the frequency at which all men, not just the middle-aged, have sexual intercourse are

- employment status
- income level
- educational level (a recent survey found, for example, that the more education you achieve, the less sex you have, a finding that nearly convinced one of my sons to quit school until I told him he could get the same results by pretending to any new girls he meets that he never finished high school—something he can fake rather easily, alas!)
- whether we own a gun or a trailer or jazz cd's (both male and female gun owners and trailer owners, as well as jazz lovers, report having more sex than we peace-loving nonhip home owners do)
- the state of our health

- the state of our partner's health
- the worries we have about our health—I know some guys, for example, who are simply petrified of anything that might increase their heart rate the least bit, and for most guys, sexual intercourse leads to a spike in heart rate, for a few seconds anyway

So take heart in knowing that for the individual, statistics about the frequency of sexual intercourse mean absolutely nothing. Maybe you will be one of the few boinking your way frequently and happily into old age.

SEX, CHICKENS, GOLF, AND DEATH

Common sense tells me, however, that for the great majority of men, the frequency of sexual intercourse is likely to decrease significantly with age. Why? For a start, most men tend to become monogamous with age, usually willingly, occasionally not, and although monogamy has much to recommend it—it is certainly easier on the nerves, for example—monogamy also breeds a sexual constancy, a certain stuck-in-the-same-way mind set and body set that can easily allow a couple's sexual relationship to be taken for granted and consequently increasingly ignored or passed over in favour of other pleasures or activities.

In that way, the history of the average couple's sex life is similar to the history of my passion for roast chicken. When I was young, you see, and had just flown my mother's coop, nothing used to fire up my taste buds as much as the smell of a newly roasted kosher capon cooking in the oven. But now that I'm older, a roasting, sweet-smelling bird no longer stimulates my salivary glands the way it once did. I do still eat lots of roast chicken, of course, especially when it's dressed in a new and beguiling manner, because there's nothing like a new spice on an old hen to whet the flagging appetite (although nature, I have been told, has not yet come up with a comparable ruse to fool a hen into thinking an old rooster is just as desirable as he used to be).

And so it is with sex, too. Thus I'm not surprised that according to a British survey, 1 in 10 seemingly happy couples between the ages of forty-five and fifty-nine admit that they abstain from sexual relations, not for religious reasons, but through an agreement that there is simply something better to do with their time. What they didn't say is what that something better is, but hey, it may be worth trying to find out.

There's more at work in aging men, however, than just constancy on the home front to temper their frequency of sexual intercourse. For example, when an aging man turns away from the pursuit of intercourse as his only goal in a sexual relationship, he is often able to develop a stronger nonsexual intimacy and bond with his partner. This improvement in his marriage increases his chances of having crucial social support later in life when he will really need it.

Also, as men get older, we need to take more time and energy to get everything working in the right order, and we are forced to invest more time and effort in doing many things that used to come much more easily. Sex is no exception. Since we have only so much energy to spare, many aging men come to the conclusion, consciously or not, that they would rather invest their limited capacities in something that is much easier to manage than sex and that on the whole is more likely to offer a positive psychological return for their effort. That's why, of course, so many middle-aged men have taken up golf.

Not only is golf the modern-day equivalent of hunting—you golf with your buddies, women are usually excluded, you (occasionally) bring back a trophy, you golf outdoors, you use clubs, and so on—but golf is also easier on the ego than sex is. After all, your golfing abilities don't tail off as you hit your middle years; no one laughs at you if you are the one with the shortest putts; if the earth moves while you're making a golf shot, you get to do it over again right away; and most important, when you golf you can really relax because you never have to worry if your partners are enjoying it as much as you are. So for many middle-aged guys, the pursuit of birdies has replaced the pursuit of birds.

What may surprise some of you, though, is that a drop-off in sex as men age may also be what nature intended. "Huh?" I can hear a few of you guys saying over that beer you've just spilled. "Why would nature be so cruel?" It may just be, you see, that less frequent sex is a way to help men live longer and better. In nearly every species, the females outlive the males, and there is some evidence that it is the male's sex drive that does us in earlier. For example, a study from the University of California at Berkeley showed that unrestrained sexual activity in adult rats led to shrinkage in spinal nerves in the male rats. Since the brain is part of the neurological system, it is conceivable that too much sex also kills some brain cells. This finding would neatly explain why guys constantly on the make are so evidently nearly brain-dead.

Of more concern, some studies have linked a higher rate of sexual activity in male animals to early death—the more sex a male has over a lifetime, the more likely he is to die younger. For example, a study on male marsupial mice who spend—I hope you're sitting down for this, guys—from five to eleven hours a day copulating (foreplay is very, very short, though) found that castrated marsupial male mice live much longer on average than the uncastrated ones.

British scientist David Gems from London's University College reviewed animal studies on sex and longevity and concluded, the *New Scientist* reports, that males of many species would outlive females if only the males could temper their sex drive. As a specific example, in nematode worms, male worms who were separated from females increased their life-spans from ten days to twenty days, double the life expectancy for the average male, as well as four days longer than the average life expectancy of female nematode worms.

The key question is: what killer effect might sexual activity exert on a male nematode worm? The most popular theory is that non-sex-seeking worms don't actually live longer, they just feel as if they've lived longer. Or, as a friend of mine suggested, perhaps they live longer just because they are nagged less. The more scientific theory is that males that don't seek sex may live longer because they tend to move around less than their sex-seeking brothers—that is, the shy guys don't spend a lot of useless energy competing with other males or defending worm territory, a theory that won't surprise anyone who has ever watched human male worms competing with each other in a singles bar. Talk about a waste of energy.

More weight to the less sex—longer life theory comes from researchers from the California Institute of Technology who recently concluded that in primates such as the mountain gorilla, in which the mating partners share at least some of the parental duties, the males seem to live nearly as long as the females. In contrast, primate males such as the chimpanzee, who play little or no role in parenting the young, tend to die significantly earlier than the females of that species. What does that have to do with sex, you are no doubt wondering. It seems to me that human males are much more like gorillas than chimpanzees (lots of women would say for sure to that), so it may pay men—they will live longer for it—to stay in family units and care for their young. The cost, as I already said, is probably less frequent, home-based sex.

Thus it may just be that a drop-off in sexual frequency with increasing age, often accompanied by a decline in the urge to have sex, may be the course that evolution has programmed to maximize a man's life expectancy. Less frequent pursuit of sex may just be healthier in the long run (although it's always wise to remember the warning of John Maynard Keynes that "in the long run, we are all dead").

Nevertheless, many men are clearly not happy with the decline in sexual energy and libido they experience as they plod into middle age, and more and more of these men are seeking out therapy for their problem. So it's time to talk about sex hormones, and what sex hormone therapy can and cannot do for you.

Testosterone—Why Men Will Always Be Boys

Testosterone is the hormone that deepens a young boy's voice, puts hair on his chest and face, and gives him his manly physique (and despite my wife's guffaws, most males do have a manly physique). In short, testosterone is what turns a male into a real man. Although it is often referred to as "the male sex hormone," all of us—men, women, and the in-between—secrete testosterone.

Testosterone starts its work early in fetal life, when it is responsible for the development of the male genitalia and the male reproductive organs, and when it is also responsible for starting that process called the masculinization of the male brain. In other words, it's fetal testosterone that has determined that a boy will want a gun in his hands as soon as he can stand and point and that will eventually produce a constant intense urge to bang some two-by-fours together to build a deck.

After birth, testosterone lies low until puberty, when a sudden huge testosterone geyser not only leads to maturation and growth of the male reproductive apparatus but also produces a change that we all dread when it rears its untamable head in adolescent boys: their sudden and intense interest in s e x. And I do mean intense. If you've ever owned one, you undoubtedly have learned that the typical adolescent boy is often nothing more than an out-of-control hormone-hijacked vehicle, and he gets little relief from those hormones even during sleep, when his wet dreams often become the cause of next-morning embarrassment for both him and his parents.

Testosterone production also rises significantly in adolescent girls, although not nearly to the same extent as it pours into pubescent boys' circulation. Why are adolescent girls also subjected to a testosterone gusher? In part because testosterone is essential to kick off two well-known phenomena: the teenage girl's sex drive, and her father's corresponding urge to buy himself a shotgun. Although most parents would rather their daughters become sexual at age forty or thereabouts, sex drive in adolescent girls is clearly an evolutionarily driven phenomenon marking their ability, and desire, to procreate.

Where Testosterone Factories Are Located and How They Function

Most testosterone is produced in the testicles, where special cells manufacture the hormone from cholesterol. Testosterone-producing cells either make their own cholesterol or grab some of the circulating cholesterol that's all around them. These days, cholesterol is usually portrayed as the guy in the black hat come to drive the life out of Dodge by plugging all the arteries in town with fat. But cholesterol is also a very necessary element of life that plays a role in many essential functions, some of which may be affected when a man unduly lowers his cholesterol count. For example, if a man allows his wife to pester him into going on a low-fat diet (the only reason most middle-aged men will ever go on a low-fat diet) and as a result his cholesterol count drops significantly, he may, according to one study, also suffer a corresponding drop in his testosterone production, which would, of course, allow his wife to boss him around even more.

A small amount of testosterone is also produced in the adrenal glands, which make it in much the same manner as the testicles do.

All the steps in testosterone synthesis are under the control of the hypothalamus, the *überstampführer* of the endocrine system. The hypothalamus discharges its duty by constantly monitoring signals from body tissues and organs that tell it how much testosterone is required for current needs. For example, if a man is getting ready to go bear hunting or in-law visiting, equivalently stressful events for most guys, he clearly needs a quick pre-emptive hit of testosterone. In anticipation, the hypothalamus secretes a chemical called gonadotropin-releasing hormone (GNRH), which heads straight to the pituitary gland and primes it to secrete luteinizing hormone (LH) and follicle-stimulating hormone (FSH). LH stimulates the testicles to produce testosterone, while FSH initiates the production of sperm—although the sperm are clearly not as necessary on a visit to the in-laws as is the extra testosterone. At least, I hope not.

Normal levels of circulating testosterone range from 300 to 1200 ng/dL (or 10.4 to 41.6 nmol/L, in SI units). Clearly, then, a man with a testosterone level of 1200 ng/dL is twice as likely to want to hunt bears and go to war as a guy with a reading of 600 ng/dL. Wrong, wrong, wrong. In fact, most doctors consider the two men to be equal in ego, aversion to in-laws, reluctance to consult a map, and need to belch and slap butt—in all those aspects central to maleness. Why? Well, since nearly all circulating testosterone travels in the blood bound to a carrier protein, circulating testosterone is relatively inactive and unavailable to the tissues (think of testosterone as one of those smallish cars that you so often see tied to the back of some oversized, cigar-shaped, highway-hogging, lawnchair-toting RV). As a result, large variations in circulating testosterone levels actually translate into little difference in "maleness"—that is, in testosterone's effects on the tissues and organs and brain.

Because of this wide range of testosterone levels, many researchers now believe that a more accurate gauge of testosterone's real effects is the level of bioavailable or unbound or "free" testosterone, which is testosterone that is not bound to a carrier protein and which is thus much more available to the tissues. A normal range of values for free testosterone is 70 to 320 ng/dL (30 to 160 pmol/L).

Unlike your commitment to your team, to your dog, or even to your true love, your testosterone level is not constant and unchanging even on a given day, and depending on when it's taken and what you are up to, the reading may vary quite a bit. Thus, the level is higher when a man is single and sinks when he hitches up. The testosterone level also falls when a man is laid off work, and as already noted, a low-fat diet may reduce testosterone level too. As a coffee lover it hurts me to say this, but at least one study found that the more coffee older women drank, the less testosterone they produced, so if you want to keep your testosterone level up, don't become an old woman, especially one who drinks coffee.

Testosterone level is also affected by the seasons—it tends to be highest in the fall and lowest in the spring—and even by the time of day (it falls during the day, rises at night—*quelle surprise*—and is highest early in the morning). Your mood and your personality also play a role. Thus, as you would expect, trial lawyers have higher testosterone levels than their nontrial colleagues. It has also been shown that a man's testosterone level tends to shoot upwards when his team wins an important match and goes down when his team loses, which explains a lot about me, I'm afraid, since the team I root for, the Chicago Cubs, hasn't won a World Series since Theodore Roosevelt was president of the United States and what's-his-name was Prime Minster of Canada.

Perhaps most important for the men reading this book, starting at around age forty, testosterone level tends to drop slowly but gradually over the ensuing years, in part because a hormone called sex-hormone-binding globulin (SHBG) begins to sop up increasing amounts of testosterone.

The rate of testosterone decline varies from man to man, however, for reasons that are still not entirely clear. Thus, according to a study from the University of Pittsburgh, Type A men (like, for example, yours truly), who are described as driven, aggressive, and combative, show a greater decline in testosterone levels with age than do their Type B "let-me-stop-to-smell-the-flowers-and-while-I'm-at-it-let-me-also-take-a-nap-in-the-flower-bed-cuz-it's-just-such-a-doo-da-great-world" brothers.

This same study also found that the more a man smokes over a lifetime and the lower his dietary fat intake, the more his testosterone level tends to fall. Surprisingly, however, in this study, weight and alcohol intake were not found to make much difference in testosterone levels.

But as noted earlier, free testosterone may be a more important measure than testosterone. So what happens to free testosterone with age? Research done by Dr. John Morley at Saint Louis University, and by others, has shown significant drops in free testosterone (as well as in the adrenal hormone dehydroepiandrosterone sulphate, or DHEAS) as males age. Morley's studies conclude that half of all men between the ages of fifty and seventy have free testosterone levels below the lowest level seen in healthy men between the ages of twenty and forty.

Why Don Cherry Has a Female Side Too

When it hits the tissues, testosterone must first get converted to other hormones, such as 5-alpha-dihydrotestosterone, which do the actual masculinizing work on the tissues. It may come as a surprise to learn that one of the hormones to which testosterone is converted—I don't know how to break this gently, guys—is estrogen. Now that's a conversion that would make even my rabbi proud, and what it means is that Jean-Claude Van Damme, Saddam Hussein, WWF stars, even Don Cherry—every man, whether he chooses to recognize his feminine side or whether he is so scared of it that he is at all times determined to impress us with his over-the-top masculinity—has some estrogen circulating in his bloodstream. And this estrogen is very important because this "female" hormone apparently helps the sperm to mature. "So what else is new?" asked a female friend of mine when I told her this bit.

Also, and this is not going to shock anyone who's ever seen a seventy-year-old man's breasts jiggle as he takes his shirt off ("Not to mention certain fifty-year-olds too," says my unforgiving wife; how does she know so much about other men taking off their shirts, I wonder), the rate of conversion of testosterone to estrogen goes up with age. It also increases with the amount of fat tissue you have managed to store because fat cells produce lots of estrogen. Since testosterone is broken down by the liver, estrogenic effects are also increased by any process that damages liver cells and hinders that breakdown process, such as excessive alcohol intake.

Why Hunters Are Hairy, Lonely, and Bald

Before I discuss testosterone's best-known jobs, its central role in the sexual arena and on the brain, let me first mention some of testosterone's other, equally important functions. Testosterone is necessary for the development and maturation of muscles, meaning that an adequate testosterone level is crucial in maintaining body mass as well as body weight. That is also why lean body mass declines with age and falling testosterone level. Testosterone is also essential for the production of sebum and for hair growth in certain areas, such as the armpits, face, and lower pubis. In addition, testosterone affects bone mass (low testosterone levels are linked to a higher risk of osteoporosis), blood cells (testosterone speeds up the production of red cells), nitrogen balance, calcium balance, carbohydrate metabolism (a low level of testosterone may increase the risk of Type II diabetes—see Chapter 5), and electrolyte balance.

Some researchers have also postulated that a low testosterone level may be a risk factor for the development of rheumatoid arthritis, perhaps because testosterone plays a role in inhibiting inflammation and cartilage erosion. Testosterone has also been shown to affect visual spatial skills and perceptual abilities. An interesting study in rats has suggested that testosterone might be more effective in preventing Alzheimer's disease than estrogen, thus raising the very scary prospect of postmenopausal women being advised to take testosterone. Some of us are just not ready for that. In fact, too much testosterone can produce unwanted physical effects (which is much more noticeable in women) such as increased facial hair, oily skin, deepening of the voice, acne, and male-pattern baldness, as well as depression and irritability —but what woman would not become depressed and irritable if she suddenly became bald, developed a beard and acne, and started singing bass in the church choir?

There is still quite a bit of controversy about testosterone's effects on the heart. For many years, it had generally been held that since being male seemed to carry a large increased risk of heart attack or stroke, testosterone must somehow be linked to that raised risk, most likely through a deleterious effect on the levels of blood lipids such as HDL (high-density lipoprotein—the good cholesterol) and LDL (low-density lipoprotein—the bad cholesterol).

Some experts now argue, however, that this testosterone–heart attack link is a spurious cause-and-effect connection on a par with the claim that drinking milk leads to a higher risk of drug use since all drug addicts drank milk in huge amounts when they were younger. Why the reassessment? First, we now know that postmenopausal women who don't take hormones are just as likely to suffer heart disease as are men. Second, if high testosterone levels really caused an increased number of heart attacks, then the rate of heart attack in men should drop significantly as men get older and their testosterone levels drop, which is the opposite of what happens. Some experts now believe that a low testosterone level might even predispose a man to a higher risk of heart attack. This issue clearly needs much more research.

In the reproduction arena, testosterone's best-known responsibility is to act as the foreman in the assembly-line production of sperm, a major responsibility to be sure, since the average male is said to produce over 100 million sperm a day, an enormous waste of effort given that nearly every one of those little guys is destined to die a quick death either at home or on some foreign battlefield, unused and unlamented.

Testosterone is also responsible for male sexual development, especially the growth of the penis at puberty, as well as for the development of secondary male sexual characteristics, such as hair growth, deepening of the voice, and pelvis development. Without testosterone, we would all be female, which, despite what the Henry Higginses of the world might tell you, would not be such a bad thing. The world would then be much less likely to suffer wars or put up with wife-beating sports stars earning multimillions of dollars, although the price would be intense disputes over splitting of restaurant bills and first use of designer outfits, as well as an overload of kitchen and bathroom renovations (has any man ever walked into his home and declared, "Honey, I think the bathroom needs redoing because those fixtures are just too old-fashioned"?).

As has already been noted, testosterone also masculinizes brain tissue, starting very early in fetal development. Thus, with the exception of only a few die-hard nonbelievers, we all now realize that there is a great deal of difference between a male infant and a female infant and that much of that difference stems from genetic factors that are simply beyond the parents', or even society's and advertising's, control.

Perhaps the clearest evidence of this difference can be seen if you offer a young boy a doll to play with. Although a few boys will undoubtedly do what nearly all young girls do with the doll, that is, construct some fairy-tale world in which the doll plays a central, and usually a very romantic, role, the typical young boy—even if he has been brought up without television and in a family fervently committed to spiritualism, pacifism (unless you attack our family), and saving of the whales, the spotted owls, liberals, and other endangered species—will inevitably point the doll at the nearest bystander and yell, "Bang, bang, you're dead." Quieter boys may instead sit there and try to tear the head off the doll to see what's inside, but then they will point it and yell, "Bang, bang, you're dead."

Social factors undoubtedly play an important role in the development of these different behaviour patterns, but much of the difference between boys and girls is also attributable to the effect of gender-specific hormones on these youngsters' brains and emotions. The problem is that we still don't know much about how these sex hormones affect us, and much of what we thought we knew may not be accurate. It has traditionally been held, for example, that testosterone leads men to be much more aggressive and violent. Thus, when injected with testosterone, lab animals tend to become more aggressive towards their cell mates as well as towards their handlers, trying to bite the fingers off the injector's hand, for example, when they are not busy trying to mount the hand, that is. In addition, prisoners incarcerated for violent crimes have been shown to have higher testosterone levels than the nonprison population. Even female prisoners with higher testosterone levels tend to exhibit more aggressive behaviour in prison than do their female convict sisters with lower levels of testosterone, and this aggressive behaviour tends to decrease as their testosterone levels fall with age. But more recent research has indicated that testosterone may be getting a bad rap, and that aggression and its ugly sibling, violence, may be linked more to estrogen receptors in the brain. In other words, it may be only when testosterone is converted to estrogen that it produces an increased tendency to become aggressive and violent. The political implications of these findings are too much for this man to contemplate.

Testosterone also affects mood and temperament. A study from Iowa found that men with low testosterone levels had an incidence of mood-and-anxiety disorders that was three times as high as that of men with normal levels. And a study from the University of California on men with low testosterone levels who had described themselves as edgy, irritable, and angry found that after several months men who were given testosterone injections now described themselves as less angry and agitated as well as happier and more optimistic (although I suspect that a good part of the reason these men were so much happier after the therapy was that they were also having more sex than they had before the injections).

A low testosterone level, then, does not make for a happy man.

Nor, however, does a high testosterone level. The Massachusetts Male Aging Study found that men with higher levels of testosterone are unhappier and lonelier than men who have lower levels. Why? Because not only have high-testosterone men been found to be more aggressive, competitive, and assertive than men with normal and low testosterone levels, they are also much more likely to be "highly interested" in sports, meaning that they probably spend a lot of time alone on the couch watching sports on TV; to be dominant; to be distant and unsympathetic; and to throw temper tantrums. They are also less likely to get married and more likely to get divorced if they do hitch up. It should be no surprise, then, that high-testerone men are also reported to get less emotional support from family and friends than do their less aggressive brothers.

Men with high testosterone levels are also probably much more likely to stray—at least that's what high testosterone levels do to the male junco bird. The higher a male junco's testosterone levels, the more likely this normally monogamous bird is to covet a junco female he has not known before, and as with juncos, so with humans, I'm sure.

So a high testosterone level does not make for a happy man either.

All in all, then, it seems that any abnormal testosterone level, whether it's too high or too low, leads men to feel worse, to have more mood swings, and to have poorer social relationships.

TESTOSTERONE AND SEXUAL FUNCTIONING

Which finally brings us to the issue that has probably kept most of you reading this far: what about testosterone and sex? How does testosterone, either the endogenous kind, which we make on our own, or the exogenous kind, which is injected or ingested or patched on, affect sex drive, sexual abilities, and the bottom line—frequency of intercourse? The answer is not nearly as simple as you might imagine, because sexual functioning in men is much more complicated than it might seem.

Now I know that to the unsophisticated (read: most women), nearly every man seems a hopelessly simple sexual being, an automatonic unrebellious slave to an overexercised imagination and overprimed, ever ready, perpetual-motion pump, driven by excessive gobs of testosterone. And I am sure that some men are like that. Most are not, however. In most guys, testosterone is only one part of what makes us tick sexually. To quote Dr. John Morley, "Sexual activity in men is composed of both libido and potency. Libido consists of sexual desire and drive, thoughts, fantasies, satisfaction and pleasure. Potency consists of the ability to obtain and maintain an erection and to ejaculate. Although potency and libido are interdependent, in men sex hormones appear to be predominantly involved in the production of libido." In other words, although testosterone does play some role in the ability to get the apparatus up and working, it plays a much more important role in producing the urge to plunge that apparatus into play in the first place, which is why testosterone is probably the reason that men think about sex so much more often than women do.

A man with a very low testosterone level has little sexual desire and is not easily aroused by appropriate sexual stimuli, which for a normal guy is usually simply the smell or sight of a nearby available person of the sex he desires, or even on occasion, a facsimile of same. A man with a very low testosterone level has fewer erections, gets less hard less often, stays hard for a shorter period of time, has fewer nighttime erections (a very good measure of a man's ability to have an erection), has a smaller volume of ejaculate, and even ejaculates less forcefully than men with higher testosterone levels. It's important to note, however, that men with even very low testosterone levels can still get aroused by sufficiently strong stimuli, such as the smell of a new Porsche, and can perform up to par as well, although I suppose the number of strokes in par is often a matter of dispute.

To summarize testosterone's role in sexual desire and drive, then, one can say that when testosterone levels are low, men don't think about sex as often; even if they think about it, they don't feel like it; and even if they feel like it, they often can't do it as well. But in the end, they can often still deliver the goods.

Testosterone-Replacement Therapy—More Bang for the Buck?

As anyone with an interest in these matters can attest, increasing numbers of experts are popping up on TV screens and in print urging all middle-aged and older men to get their testosterone levels measured, and if the level is at all "low," to start taking testosterone-replacement therapy. After all, these experts ask, if it does nothing else, wouldn't this exogenous source of testosterone improve every man's sexual functioning? I'm afraid it's not that simple.

We know that many men with abnormally low testosterone levels respond well to testosterone-replacement therapy. They have more energy, their mood is raised, their sexual functioning improves. In fact, these guys with abnormally low testosterone levels are the ones who make up a disproportionately high percentage of all the happy hangers who are always trotted forth in uncontrolled studies and anecdotal reports that tout the benefits of testosterone-replacement therapy.

But middle-aged men with abnormally low testosterone levels make up only a small percentage of all middle-aged men. What about the much more substantial number of men who have the symptoms that some experts typically ascribe to andropause but whose testosterone levels are normal or even "low normal"? These symptoms include:

- mood swings
- fatigue
- difficulties in concentrating
- increased anxiety levels
- physical aches and pains
- low libido
- decreased strength
- poorer memory

Some experts have recently claimed that this constellation of symptoms constitutes a new syndrome known as partial androgen deficiency in the aging male, or PADAM (best to say that with drum roll), or ADAM, androgen deficiency in the aging male. Both these acronyms describe that cohort of men with low-normal testosterone levels who suffer symptoms such as lower energy levels, mood changes, and sexual slowdown and who may as a result of their falling testosterone levels also be more likely to develop some of the diseases traditionally ascribed to hormonal changes with age, such as osteoporosis, muscle loss, and perhaps even heart disease.

So what should PADAM guys do, if they actually exist? That's easy. The first thing they should do is what we should all probably be doing whether our testosterone levels are low or not—we should keep those levels up naturally. How do you do that? Exercise, sleep, compete, and eat meat. According to an article in *Men's Health*, studies have revealed that testosterone levels are higher in weight lifters and serious competitors and higher in meat eaters than in vegetarians, while testosterone levels tend to drop in men who overexercise and don't sleep that much. My wife, by the way, lifts weights, eats meat, and often sleeps in, and you would never want to face her over a gin rummy hand. That explains just about everything you need to know about me.

If the natural methods don't work, however, you are left with only two choices: doing nothing or taking testosterone-replacement therapy. So what can testosterone replacement therapy do for you? For a start, it will increase your sexual desire. It does that for everyone, even for many postmenopausal women who are given testosterone to boost their sexual interest and response. On the down side, however, these women also report a sudden intense urge to buy a set of Craftsman tools, but hey, those tools last a lifetime. Or so my handymen tell me. As a typical Jewish man, you see, I have no tools—only a set of phone numbers of tradesmen to call for estimates.

What is not nearly as clear, however, is whether testosterone-replacement therapy is necessary or even desirable for those other symptoms you have, which may simply be normal components of aging or which may be due to other problems—depression, for example. The studies that could tell us which of those symptoms are caused by abnormally low hormone levels and, more important, which men should take hormones to alleviate their symptoms have simply not been done yet, and many researchers believe that the move to categorize most of those vague symptoms into a new syndrome is nothing more than an attempt to medicalize the normal and inevitable changes of aging.

This unsettled debate leaves much room for speculation, and many doctors and self-styled experts have leaped into the breach with books and articles detailing the miracles you will experience if you just follow their advice. So as a leaping doctor, what do I think, you would no doubt like to know.

I do agree that some low-testosterone men are suffering from such a syndrome and that some would benefit from testosterone-replacement therapy. Where I disagree with many of the hormone hucksters is in their belief that *all* men with lowered levels of testosterone should be taking testosterone-replacement therapy. To me, this is jump-starting your gun, and that is not enough. To start, as I said about menopause, I am reluctant to support the medicalization of a condition that has not yet been shown to be a pathological disease. We must tread very warily when we consider treating *symptoms* with potent drugs. Further, those diseases that are being touted as preventable with testosterone-replacement therapy, such as osteoporosis and heart disease, are probably in most cases equally preventable with proper lifestyle adjustment, and any effort to push hormones would deflect attention and resources away from prevention—to me, a much more important focus for health experts and for patients themselves. Thus, I believe that if you wish to prevent osteoporosis, you will be doing yourself much more of a favour if you increase the amount of exercise you do instead of relying on hormones.

In addition, as I said earlier, it's possible, perhaps even probable, that a lower though still normal testosterone level and its corresponding decrease in sexual drive might just be an evolutionary manipulation to allow an aging man a better chance to live longer and better by ensuring that he stops fighting younger bucks for territory and younger, fertile mates.

Also, since men with lower testosterone levels report getting more emotional support from friends and family than do their more aggressive brothers, perhaps as we get older lower testosterone levels increase our chances of having better social relationships, which are known to decrease the risk of premature death in older men. Maybe lower testosterone levels work to keep men at home, where they can concentrate on improving their familial relationships and protecting their DNA-bearing offspring (although to be fair, a man can never really tell, can he, which of those heavy eaters on his couch bears his DNA and which one is an accidental tourist, and besides, most of those heavy eaters do not want or need to be protected). What's more, because of the feedback loop that testosterone is part of, any outside source of testosterone is likely to affect other hormone levels as well. In one study, for example, middle-aged men who took testosterone all experienced a drop in follicle-stimulating hormone, luteinizing hormone, and sex-hormone-binding globulin. Researchers simply don't know yet what these changes mean.

The most important reason for going slow on testosterone replacement therapy, though, is the very important concern about prostate disease and prostate cancer. Several studies have linked higher testosterone levels not only to prostate enlargement but also to prostate cancer. Given that prostate cancer is the most common cancer in elderly gents, any potential increased risk from testosterone-replacement therapy in younger men is a serious concern indeed. Clearly, much better studies are needed to tell us that messing with nature in this way will not make matters worse.

Until those studies are done, however, is there a formula to help you decide if you should consider testosterone-replacement therapy? I'm afraid not. The advice here is no different from what doctors tell women who ask about hormone-replacement therapy for menopause: you have to answer this one for yourself. If you think you have a problem, you should first get a physical exam and get your testosterone and free testosterone levels measured. If your levels are low, you must weigh your risks, your symptoms, your beliefs, your family history, your worries, and your partner's concerns. You must also add in what you expect the hormone therapy to accomplish, and then you will have some idea about what's right for you. Thus, men who have low free testosterone levels and who have endured sudden and intense changes that interfere with their ability to function or to enjoy life—and especially if they are also found to be at risk for osteoporosis—are more likely to decide to use testosterone-replacement therapy and to benefit from it. In contrast, men who have vague symptoms of fatigue, loss of libido, and occasional mood swings and who have a strong family history of prostate cancer are unlikely to choose that course, nor should they. If, in the end, you do opt to try testosterone-replacement therapy anyway, keep a close watch on your prostate (you don't actually have to watch it yourself; that might be difficult to do, so get someone else to do it for you).

CHAPTER 4

The Prostate—Or the Terminator, Because It Gets All Men in the End

The dog and the human are the only two mammals
whose prostates give them trouble. Could that be because they're
also the most domesticated animals?

—Dr. Martin Gleave, urologist

I have three standard speeches in my public-speaking repertoire, each of which has been given a fond though sarcastic nickname by members of my family. The speech I give most often describes strategies for adopting a healthier lifestyle, a speech I call "Healthy Lifestyle—Myth or Reality?" My son Tim, who once heard me give this talk three times in one week, calls it the "s.o.s." speech, "because," he told me after sitting through the third rendition, "it's the same old shit every time, Dad." That boy has a career as a lawyer in front of him, I think, or perhaps as an editorial writer. The second speech I often give carries the title "Menopause—The Best Years." My wife, however, a woman of a certain age, has dubbed this speech "Menopause—Or Hey! Turn the Bloody Heat Down, I'm Boiling Here." And finally, there is my favourite and most requested talk, the one that I call "The Prostate—An Owner's Manual" and that my wife has renamed "The Terminator, Because It Gets All Men in the End."

I'm afraid that she's dead right. The prostate does indeed get nearly every man in the end. The prostate is the "ha-ha, you're it" gland, the gender leveller, the even-upper, that little gland that squarely pays us men back for all those years during which we wondered and frequently scoffed at our partner's and female friends' often relentless struggles with periods, pregnancies, PMS, postpartum pits, and all those other hormonal and glandular changes to which women are biologically captive.

As the years go by, however, it is practically inevitable that the prostate will force itself into an aging man's unwilling consciousness. For many men, the prostate eventually becomes the body part he mournfully rues the most as he stands sleepily jiggling in that Hebraic shaking-prayer stance in front of his toilet at five A.M., having been jolted awake for the second or third time by pressure from his bladder, waiting impatiently for that weak yellow ribbon to begin its slow trickle and remembering when he could go without going for over ten hours, and when he could still hit a tree or a zucchini plant from a distance of at least five yards. Now he can hardly hit the toilet bowl that lies immediately below him, a fact that his partner, and the telltale dried-up spots on the bathroom floor, regularly remind him of.

What Is a Prostate and Where Can You Find One?

The prostate is a small gland that's part of the male genitourinary system, the main player in both urinary and genital functions. When a man is young, the prostate is not a big guy, invariably described as walnut-sized or the size of a large strawberry, certainly not large at all when compared with organs such as the liver and spleen. Even when it grows or enlarges, a process called benign hyperplasia, the prostate doesn't become much bigger than a large apricot. Doctors, by the way, as I'm sure you've noticed, are the most imagination-challenged people on earth; the only things we ever compare organs or tissues with are fruits and veggies and the occasional nut.

Now the reason it's important to explain how large a prostate may become is that if the prostate were merely the average body part, size wouldn't matter, just as size doesn't really matter for the other important parts of a male's sexual apparatus. ("Such as his brain," my wife suggests.) For the prostate, however, as for a semidetached bungalow, location is destiny. It's where the prostate has chosen to set up shop that makes it such a problem-filled gland. The prostate, you see, is located directly below the bladder, where it just happens to surround the urethra, the tube through which urine and semen must pass on their way to the breathlessly awaiting world.

This location leads to two problems for the average male. The first and more minor of these is that a prostate cannot be felt through the

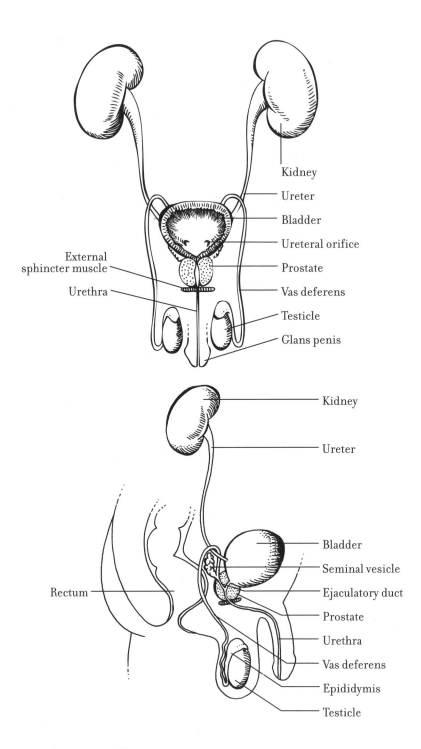

MALE GENITOURINARY SYSTEM

top frontal view; *bottom* side view

Adapted from *The Intelligent Patient Guide to Prostate Cancer*,
by S. Larry Goldenberg, 1992.

thick abdominal wall, which is thicker in some men than in others, of course. That means that the only way to get a good feel of the prostate, to palpate the prostate, is to put a finger into the rectum and push up. This is the digital rectal exam, or DRE (most men think that DRE actually stands for dreaded rectal exam), a procedure that most men look forward to about as much as they do to an excursion with the wife to buy a new pair of shoes. (A cute *New Yorker* cartoon: two husbands leashed side by side to topped-up parking meters in front of Bloomingdale's. Been there, by the way, and certainly felt like that.)

The second problem with the prostate's location is more serious and disturbing: when the prostate grows, it squeezes the urethra, with the consequences I shall describe below.

Do You Really Need a Prostate?

The short answer is no. After all, women do just fine without one. Men do need a prostate, however, if they want to procreate the natural way—that is, without the assistance of an in-vitro clinic that can pass on your DNA without your active participation.

The prostate helps sperm survive. You see, seminal fluid originates in the testicles, and from there it has to take a sort of sperm portage by first passing upwards through the vas deferens. From the vas, the seminal fluid passes into the prostate via structures called ejaculatory ducts. The ejaculatory ducts are a sort of way station, a Sperm Hilton, where seminal fluid can lay-by for a while before being ejected into the urethra, and finally to, well, that depends on which way you're leaning at the time.

The problem with this setup is that sperm cells are not very large guys, and to a sperm cell, that long transpenile voyage is a very trying and arduous journey. So it's not surprising that they require a rejuvenation hit on their trip. The prostate gland (along with the seminal vesicles that connect to the ejaculatory ducts) serves as the Sperm City Café; when the seminal fluid passes through, Flo and the rest of the café's waitresses top it up with added liquid as well as nutrients to help it on its suicide mission.

How the Prostate Can Change Your Life

The three most common prostate conditions are:

- infection or inflammation (prostatitis)
- benign prostatic growth (hyperplasia)
- prostate cancer

Prostatitis

Until the age of forty or so, most men can safely ignore their prostates, and nearly all of us are only too happy to do so. The exception is that guy unlucky enough to develop a prostate inflammation or infection, both of which are called prostatitis. The difference between an inflammation and an infection is that with an infection, there is a recognizable infectious agent to account for the symptoms. As many men have found out to their chagrin, however, often that agent, like a teenager when there are chores to do, cannot be easily located or isolated. With a prostate inflammation, there is no known infectious agent at work, although the process may have started as an infection and the responsible party has now fled the scene, like that broker who assured me that those Bre-X shares would go up, up, up.

Acute Bacterial Prostatitis   Acute bacterial prostate infections are happily relatively infrequent events. This infection tends to happen mainly in young men, and sadly, it's an impossible infection to ignore because acute prostatitis often explodes with many of the sudden severe symptoms that women who have had a bladder infection will instantly recognize: a burning sensation when urinating, a need to urinate often, a need to urinate NOW THIS MINUTE, and for some men the worst symptom: when they get there, they just can't go as easily as is their wont. Other symptoms may include fever, pain in either the low back or the low abdomen, and a general feeling of sickness, what my son Jonah rather accurately calls, "feeling like shit." He wants to be a doctor, so he is practising our lingo.

A bacterial infection leaves the prostate swollen and inflamed, so when it's palpated, it is tender and feels "boggy." Treatment of acute prostatitis is antibiotics in high enough doses to kill all the little buggers. Usually that means taking a lot of antibiotic, because once bacteria find their way into the prostate, they love to linger there. If you think of the prostate as a bacterial spa, warm and wet and well supplied with life-sustaining liquids, nutrients, and other bacteria to consort with, it is clear that the bacteria must be hit regularly and very hard if they are to be ousted. This usually means taking the antibiotics for a month and sometimes longer.

Chronic Bacterial Prostatitis   Chronic bacterial prostatitis is a real pain in the butt for everyone who has to deal with it, although it's clearly more of a pain for the patient than the doctor. A chronic bacterial prostate infection is generally produced by an acute infection that no longer responds to short-term use of antibiotics. Symptoms may include pain in the low back or low abdomen, as well as the need to void urgently, frequency of urination, burning on urination, and—here's the real kicker—pain on ejaculation.

But sadly, it often gets even worse than that. What can possibly be worse than pain on ejaculation, you ask? To diagnose the infection, the physician usually opts to get a sample of fluid from the prostate, and he does this via a prostatic massage, the kind of procedure that makes every man who gets one sure he's going steady with the doctor afterwards. Also, like an acute infection of the prostate or an unemployed house-guest brother-in-law, chronic bacterial infections of the prostate are hard to get rid of. Treatment consists of several weeks and often months of antibiotics, and unfortunately, the antibiotic regime must often be repeated, since this problem has a habit of recurring. Some men cannot come off the antibiotic at all because their symptoms recur as soon as they discontinue their medication.

Nonbacterial Prostatitis   Now the prostate infections I have already mentioned are not pleasant, and some are downright nasty, but if you are going to feel sorry for anyone, guys, save your pity for the bro who develops nonbacterial prostatitis. Not only is this a visitor who comes to stay, but as with that stray alley cat that came by for only one evening, two tops, and who has now become an unremovable fungus on your living room couch, there is also not a whole lot you can do to get rid of nonbacterial prostatitis when it lodges chez vous.

The symptoms of nonbacterial prostatitis are the same as for bacterial prostatitis. A whole host of possible suspects, such as *Chlamydia trachomatis* and *Mycoplasma hominis*, have been linked with a higher risk of nonbacterial prostatitis, but these organisms are also found in the urethras of males without this condition, so something else must be going on in guys who end up with nonbacterial prostatitis besides simple exposure to potentially infective organisms.

If doctors don't know what causes nonbacterial prostatitis, how do they treat it? Well, not knowing the cause of a condition has never stopped doctors from rushing in to treat it, and so it is with this baby as well. It is usually treated with antibiotics directed at the organisms that might be culpable, such as those nasty chlamydiae. Men with this condition are also advised to avoid or at least decrease their intake of substances known to make prostate symptoms worse. These include aspartame, caffeine, spicy foods, and alcohol, but as a long-time lover of coffee, pickles, chilis, wine, and Diet Coke, five of the seven essential food groups (salami and garlic are the others), I must say that if these substances do not obviously make your symptoms worse, there is no real reason to avoid them entirely.

Finally, as every person with this condition invariably asks: "So what about *it*, eh, Doc?" Good news, guys. *It* is ok. In fact, these days most specialists say that "it" should be mandatory on the theory that just as an old car needs an oil change from time to time, the prostate needs its fluids emptied regularly too, and happily you are supposed to empty your gland considerably more often than you change the oil in your car. But please don't ask me how often. Whatever you believe is right is fine by me, unless, that is, you start going blind or your hands start shaking. That's probably too often.

Prostadynia   *Prostadynia* refers to prostate-related symptoms that have no discernible cause. Quite a few guys have this complaint. These men have entirely normal physical examinations, and all the tests of their prostate, bladder, and urethra are likewise normal.

So what causes prostadynia? There are several theories. It could be that men with prostadynia are harbouring an as-yet-unidentified pathogen; it could be that their symptoms are caused by some kind of neurological dysfunction—that these guys are just supersensitive to normal stimuli emanating from that area; or it could be that this condition is a muscular ache—the equivalent of a tension headache around the prostate; or it might just be a psychological condition, some kind of glorious prostate obsession.

To treat the symptoms of prostadynia, avoid the usual suspects—caffeine, alcohol, spices, aspartame. Nonsteroidal anti-inflammatory drugs, alpha-blockers such as terazocin, and an army of other medications may also be helpful. It is also essential to try to take your mind off your behind, easier for me to advise than for you to do, of course.

Benign Prostatic Hyperplasia
For most men, the prostate grows with age. And grows. And grows. Thus, a man who lives to age sixty has a 50 per cent chance of suffering

from an enlarged prostate, or benign prostatic hyperplasia, and if he is lucky enough to live into his mid-eighties, he has a 90 per cent chance of suffering from an enlarged prostate. Not every enlarged prostate requires treatment, however. It's only when an enlarged prostate causes symptoms significant enough to interfere with its owner's life or when it grows large enough to produce potentially significant medical complications that its owner requires therapy. The common estimate is that one in four men requires treatment for benign prostatic hyperplasia by the age of eighty, but that also means that three in four do not, something to comfort you tonight on your second post-midnight voiding expedition.

Why the prostate grows is not clear. Hormones, especially testosterone, must play a key role, but most studies have been unable to find a consistent link between testosterone levels and prostate size. Most experts also believe that environmental influences play a role in making the prostate swell, although again, studies have failed to nail down consistent patterns between environmental factors and prostate size.

Symptoms   *Prostatism* refers to the complex of symptoms produced by an enlarged prostate, which include most prominently:

- having to get up at night to urinate, sometimes several times
- a slower and weaker urine flow
- a feeling that the bladder has not been completely emptied after a visit to the can
- a need to urinate more often
- a sense of urgency, so that when you gotta go, you really gotta go
- dribbling, although this is clearly not the same kind of dribbling you associate with Michael Jordan

The American Urological Association grades these symptoms on a scale of one (mild) to five (will-no-one-rid-me-of-this-gland?), and the higher the overall score, the more likely it is that therapy will offer some relief.

Do not, however, assume that if you develop the symptoms listed above, you are merely suffering from benign prostatic hyperplasia. You must see your doctor to ensure that these symptoms are not the first sign of prostate cancer, a prostate infection, or a nonurological problem. (To be accurate, you don't actually "see" the doctor while he or she is checking your prostate, but if you do, the Cirque du Soleil would like to give you an audition.) For example, some men who complain about having to get up at night to pee are not suffering from benign prostatic hyperplasia but rather from some type of sleep disturbance, particularly sleep apnea (see Chapter 7), and they only get up so often to pee because their sleep is disturbed by the sleep apnea. In other words, although the cart may be the need to urinate, the horse is actually the sleep disorder.

Is there any reason to treat benign prostatic hyperplasia that is not causing significant symptoms? The occasional large prostate can cause complications that require urgent medical intervention, such as a sudden inability to urinate or recurrent bladder infections, without having betrayed its presence with significant symptoms, but that is not common. For the vast majority of men who house a larger prostate, it's not the size but the symptoms that determine the need for therapy, and even a large prostate does not require surgery if the symptoms remain mild. One study found that over four years of observation, the majority of patients with mild symptoms of benign prostatic hyperplasia did not go on to suffer severe symptoms. Another study compared men who opted for early surgery with men who chose watchful waiting for their benign prostatic hyperplasia (the doctor was watchful, the patient was waiting) and found that only 24 per cent of the latter group required surgery over the seven years of the study.

Treatment   Saw palmetto, a herb that is widely used in Europe for benign prostatic hyperplasia, is commonly said to relieve symptoms. Unfortunately, no good double-blind studies have been done on this herb, so for now, the rallying cry of most conservative doctors is "Buyer beware," just as it should be "Buyer beware" for all the drugs those more conservative doctors give you as well. As for me, when I get there —and it's not too far away, I'm afraid—I will certainly saw the palmetto first. I'm not that conservative yet.

Finasteride, a drug that's known as a 5-alpha reductase inhibitor, can help slow the progression of benign prostatic hyperplasia and quell symptoms by slowing down the breakdown of testosterone to its more active metabolites. Several other drugs known as alpha-blockers (terazocin, prazocin, doxazocin, and others) have also been shown to reduce the symptoms of benign prostatic hyperplasia by relaxing muscle fibres in the prostate. To varying degrees, all these drugs improve symptoms such as the need to urinate at night or the feeling that the bladder is not completely emptied after a visit to the can. They also improve what urologists refer to as "peak flow rate," meaning that the tiny tinny trickle through a tense and thickened prostate is somewhat enhanced.

Like all drugs, however, these medications produce side effects. Among the side effects to be expected on finasteride, decreased libido and impotence stand out, as they usually do, whereas dizziness is often the main problem with alpha-blockers—not too surprising when you learn that in the past these drugs were used primarily to lower blood pressure.

Placebos also have a great track record with this condition. In many studies, placebos worked nearly as well as the expensive drugs did, and they even produced side effects not unlike those produced by the medications. For example, in one study the placebos worked so well that the men who had been taking them still claimed an improvement in their symptoms two years after the study had stopped. In fact, the placebo takers were so happy with the ersatz medication that they refused to give it up even when the study had ended and they were told that the pills contained nothing but sugar. Now these are guys with whom I would love to discuss my Bre-X shares.

When your symptoms are severe enough, you must turn to surgery. Several types of surgery are available. In fact, you can think of a urologist's office as a kind of shopping channel, where you get more choices to purchase something you don't really want than you had ever imagined possible. The old standby for prostate surgery is usually referred to rather unkindly but not at all inaccurately as a Roto-Rooter job, although the official term is *transurethral resection of the prostate*, or TURP. In this procedure, the surgeon pushes his instruments into the prostate by way of the urethra, and then he hacks away. At least, that's the way most patients view a TURP, although to be fair, urologists see it somewhat more benignly—but then they have a better, and less painful, seat in the stands to view it from.

As a potential improvement on the old hack-and-slash method, some surgeons believe in burning the tissue with an electric current or a laser, or they—hold on to your seats, guys—microwave the tissue with a new gadget called a Prostatron, although if I were having this done on me, I would want strict guarantees that the instrument would not start to arc in there. The latest inclusion in the prostate surgery

arsenal is a procedure known as TUNA, for transurethral needle abla-
tion, in which a catheter with electrodes attached to its end is inserted
into the prostate via the urethra. With the catheter in place, the
urologist lets loose a radio frequency through the electrodes, which not
only kills the tissue around it but, if you're really lucky, picks up the
Howard Stern show at the same time. Well, better that than country-
and-western music.

Prostate Cancer
What do actor Roger Moore, General Norman Schwartzkopf, former
French president François Mitterand, failed presidential candidate
Bob Dole, Phi Beta Crappa alumnus Frank Zappa, Washington, D.C.,
mayor and convicted felon Marion Barry, and Iran's ex-Supreme
leader Ayatollah Khomeini have in common? Yes, they all either are
has-beens or are dead, but the other link between them is that they
also all have, or had, prostate cancer. Prostate cancer is an equal-
opportunity cancer that can strike any man. Although everyone knows
that women have a one-in-nine chance of getting breast cancer if they
live long enough, too few people know that middle-aged men stand a
one-in-eleven chance of developing a clinically significant prostate
cancer if we live long enough, and that 3 per cent of us will eventually
die from prostate cancer.

After skin cancer, prostate cancer is the most common cancer
affecting men in nearly every developed country, and, after lung
cancer, prostate cancer is the second leading cause of deaths from
cancer in men in the Western world. Prostate cancer accounts for 32
per cent of cancers in North American men and 14 per cent of deaths
from cancer. What is particularly alarming is that the number of cases
of prostate cancer is increasing in frequency as more and more of us
sunshine boys live to a ripe old age, although at least some of that
increase must be attributed to better diagnostic abilities, as well as to
a huge growth in the number of frightened men like me who have run
off to get themselves tested for prostate cancer.

Risk Factors   What do researchers know about the causes of prostate
cancer? Lots, but not nearly enough.

First, we know that age is a very important risk factor. Nine to 10
per cent of men will be diagnosed with prostate cancer by the time they
hit the age of seventy-five, and after that the older we get, the higher

our risk. Race too plays an important role; North American black men have twice the risk of North American white men. Testosterone also plays an important role in prostate cancer. But the relationship between testosterone and prostate cancer is much like the one between my mother and me—much more complicated than it seems on the surface. For a start, researchers have known for many years that prostate cancer cells need testosterone to grow. In addition, some studies have linked higher rates of prostate cancer to higher levels of testosterone and free testosterone, although the Massachusetts Male Aging Study did not find such a link. Moreover, a study from Duke University found that men with small shoulder spans in relation to the rest of their bodies—someone like yours truly—also seem to have a higher risk of prostate cancer. Ever since I read that, by the way, I've been walking around with my chest puffed out and with my shoulders held back as far as they'll go. Unfortunately for me, however, shoulder span is not linked to cancer risk by the way you stand but more likely by the way testosterone affects body build as you are growing. That is, the influence that testosterone exerts on your risk of prostate cancer may be set very early in life, and so measuring testosterone levels later in life may not reflect testosterone's real effects on the prostate.

Family history is also important in determining your risk of prostate cancer. About 9 to 10 per cent of all prostate cancers are estimated to be caused by genetic predisposition. Thus, a man who has a first-degree male relative (father, brother, grandfather) who has had prostate cancer is two to three times as likely as his peers to develop prostate cancer himself, and the younger the relative was when he developed the cancer, the higher this man's risk. A man with two first-degree relatives who had prostate cancer has an eight- to tenfold increased risk himself. Familial prostate cancers also tend to occur more frequently in younger men, and they also tend to be more aggressive cancers. As a result, most experts advise men with a family history of prostate cancer to get tested for the disease much sooner than the average guy, probably from the age of forty on (see the section on diagnosis, below).

There is also some evidence that a man's risk of prostate cancer goes up if his mother's family has a strong history of this tumour, and just to scare you completely, there may also be a slight increase in colon and breast cancers in such families.

A few years ago, a highly publicized study claimed to have discovered a link between vasectomies at a young age (under thirty-five) and an increased risk of prostate cancer. Most other studies have failed to confirm this link, however, and the consensus seems to be that even if a vasectomy does raise the risk of prostate cancer, it results in a very negligible increase (although I must admit, as a typical male, that "negligible increased risk" is an oxymoron when it comes to men and genital-area cancers). Thus, most experts agree that for most men the benefits of a vasectomy far outweigh the slight possibility of an increased risk for prostate cancer.

Environmental and dietary factors also play a large role in this tumour. Although microscopic evidence for the presence of prostate cancer is fairly constant in men throughout the world, the rates at which prostate cancers grow to cause trouble vary significantly in different areas of the world. For example, Chinese men living in China have among the lowest rates of death from prostate cancer in the world. But when Chinese men move to North America, their risk of death from prostate cancer goes up, and within two generations the rates for their offspring are much closer to those for other men born in North America. Not only do similar patterns hold for just about any group that has been examined, but there is also clear evidence now that prostate cancer rates are gradually rising in all those countries that are steadily becoming westernized.

So, you may be wondering, of all the most significant westernizing influences—drugs, sex, TV talk shows, and bowling—which ones are responsible for this rising tide of prostate cancers? None of the above, I'm afraid. The fault lies elsewhere, dear brutes, although it doesn't seem to lie with heavy drinking or smoking, neither of which has, alas, been linked to an increased risk of prostate cancer.

Rather, the guiltiest party is probably diet. A diet high in saturated fat, especially if the fats are derived from red meat and dairy products, has been correlated with a higher risk of prostate cancer and a worsening of an already existing malignancy as well. In addition, a study on mice showed that switching the mice to a significantly lower fat diet, from 40 per cent to 21 per cent fat, could slow and perhaps even stop the growth of their prostate cancers, although as I've already cautioned, a diet too low in fat may reduce one's level of testosterone and thus lead to other unpleasant ramifications, such as the lead role in *Evita*. I'm happy to say, though, that Dr. Dean Ornish, who opened our eyes to the effect that a low-fat diet and other lifestyle modifications could have in reversing established heart disease, is currently doing a study to see what effect a very low-fat diet combined with stress reduction and regular exercise might have on prostate cancer. The first results should be available about a year from now.

Other studies have found that the risk of prostate cancer might be lowered by a high intake of lycopene, an antioxidant in the carotene family. Lycopene is found in watermelon, red grapefruit, and some shellfish, but by far the largest doses are in tomatoes, especially cooked tomatoes. In a study of health professionals, three of the four foods found to be associated most strongly with a lower risk of prostate cancer were tomato sauce, tomatoes, and pizza, although I must say that I am just a tad suspicious when a study headed by a man with an Italian background finds that we would all be better off if we ate more pizza. By the way, the reason that cooked tomatoes are better for your prostate than raw ones is that cooking breaks down the lycopene and allows it to be more easily absorbed.

Other vitamins seem to play a large role in preventing prostate cancer as well.

- For example, a very hopeful recent study found that men who were smokers and who took daily supplements of 50 mg of vitamin E, a low supplemental dose compared with the ones used in most other studies, reduced their risk of prostate cancer by over 30 per cent and their risk of dying from prostate cancer by over 40 per cent.
- A study of fifteen thousand Harvard doctors found that those who had the highest blood levels of beta-carotene had the lowest rates of prostate cancer.
- Vitamin D also appears to be an important factor. It is known, for example, that in more northern countries, where people have less exposure to sunlight than in other parts of the world (sunlight promotes the body's production of vitamin D), men have higher rates of prostate cancer. As well, a study done on rats at the University of Pittsburgh found that high doses of vitamin D helped shrink advanced prostate cancers and also lowered the number of metastases.
- Some researchers believe that a deficiency in folic acid may also be a potential risk factor.
- And at least one study has found that a fibre-rich diet is also linked to a lower risk of prostate cancer.

The upshot of all this, then, is that to try to prevent prostate cancer, you should be eating more grains, fibre, fruits, and veggies (especially pizza), and you should perhaps also be taking some supplemental vitamin E. But before you decide to do that, read Chapter 6.

Finally, the factor you have all no doubt been waiting for me to discuss: intercourse. This one is still a subject of much controversy, although a well-done study did find, I'm afraid, that men who have more frequent intercourse have a higher risk of prostate cancer. But soft, my pals, because there is a small rope of hope to cling to, thin though that thread may be. You see, this finding does not establish a cause-and-effect relationship between frequency of intercourse—or probably more accurately, ejaculation—and prostate cancer. It may just be that the hormones (and other factors) that drive certain men to adopt a philosophy of "Damn the torpedoes! I've got to empty my load, no matter what the consequences!" may also be what condemns such men to a higher risk of prostate cancer. For the average guy, it appears doubtful that slowing down the rate at which you do it will lower your risk of prostate cancer, so full steam ahead, and may God be with you. You're welcome.

One last note: although I, along with most other middle-aged guys, tend to make a lot of bad jokes about prostate disease and prostate cancer, in large part because it is not yet a part of our lives, this disease strikes intense fear into the hearts of even the strongest men. Prostate cancer is not a laughing matter but is the source of a great deal of stress and depression. In fact, men diagnosed with prostate cancer are more likely to commit suicide than men diagnosed with any other kind of cancer.

Symptoms   Unfortunately, in its most curable stage, when it is still small and confined to the prostate, prostate cancer does not generally produce any symptoms to announce its presence. If you remember nothing else from this chapter, remember this: prostate cancer is a silent killer.

As a prostate cancer grows, it can cause symptoms similar to those associated with benign prostatic hyperplasia, and when it spreads, it will produce symptoms associated with the area it has invaded. For example, if it metastasizes to a bone, a favourite place for prostate cancer to spread to, it will cause severe pain associated with bone cancer.

Diagnosis   Prostate cancer is often compared with breast cancer—both cancers increase significantly with age; both are hormonally driven cancers; breast cancer is the second leading cause of death from cancer in women, while prostate cancer is the second leading cause of death from cancer in men; and until recently they had both been neglected for far too long by research funding agencies. But these two cancers differ in at least one vital respect: you don't ever want to diagnose prostate cancer through a self-examination.

Thus, in the diagnosis of prostate cancer, you are completely in the hand of a stranger. Unfortunately, until relatively recently, the only way to diagnose prostate cancer was through a digital rectal exam, the old one-fingered salute, a procedure that for some strange reason seems to be the butt of much urological humour. It's not unusual, for example, for a urologist to tell a whimpering, butt-up man, "You know, George, I'm not really sure what's going on up there. I think I want a second opinion." And as a joke, he pretends to get another digit ready. (This is an excellent illustration of why urologists rarely get invited to mixed parties, "mixed" meaning that there are other human beings there.)

Although I wouldn't say this to a guy fetalized on the exam table, the digital rectal exam is rather insensitive—that is, it cannot detect small tumours. Less than 40 per cent of prostate cancers detected by a digital rectal exam are still confined to the prostate, so by the time a prostate cancer is palpable with a digital rectal exam, there is a strong likelihood that it has already spread. For this reason, the digital rectal exam remains a rather poor screening tool for prostate cancer. That is why there was so much optimism about a blood test for prostate cancer, the prostate specific antigen (PSA) test, because it was hoped that the PSA would replace the digital rectal exam and serve as a useful, sensitive, and specific screening test for prostate cancer.

PSA is an enzyme produced by prostate cells that liquefies the ejaculate. Small amounts of PSA leak into the circulation and are easily measured, and since PSA is specific for prostate cells, the level of PSA in the blood is an excellent measure of prostate disease. A "normal" reading is generally less than 4.0 ng/mL, although this standard goes up a bit with age and prostate size. The trend in PSA level is also very important. Thus, a PSA level of even 4.0 would be significant in a man, especially one in middle age, who had a reading of 0.5 two years ago and 1.5 last year.

Unfortunately, PSA levels are not nearly as specific for cancer as we would like them to be, primarily because PSA levels can go up with just about anything that affects the prostate, not just cancer. Thus, the PSA level goes up after ejaculation (you have to avoid ejaculating for forty-eight hours before getting tested, not as harsh a requirement as most middle-aged guys would like you to believe it is), with benign prostatic hyperplasia, following a vigorous prostate massage, and occasionally after exercise. It can even go up following the dreaded digital derrière dilatation.

What all that means is that an elevated PSA level can indicate either a serious disease or a more benign occurrence, and happily, a majority of men with PSA levels between 4.0 and 10.0 do not have a malignancy. Invariably, however, based on the widely accepted axiom—one held in equal esteem by both a terrified patient and a malpractice-phobic physician—that all abnormal tests must be explained or else, a man with an elevated level of PSA will undergo further tests to rule out prostate cancer. There, if you excuse the expression, lies the rub, because these tests involve ultrasound of the prostate as well as multiple biopsies. Not only are these procedures emotionally traumatic—if you think the average guy feels ridiculously sorry for himself when he has a cold, wait till you see the same guy after he's been told someone is going to stick a needle into his prostate—but they are also costly. Although a prostate biopsy is called a minor procedure, it's always wise to remember that the only good definition of a minor procedure is "something that's going to be done on someone else." Moreover, even minor procedures can occasionally result in complications such as excess bleeding and infection and, rarely, neurological damage.

This is why although there is widespread acceptance of the PSA test as a good measure of follow-up after cancer therapy (the PSA level should drop into the normal range, and one should worry again only if it starts to go up), there is still controversy about using the PSA as a mass screening test on many millions of men who are healthy and have no reason to suspect they may be harbouring a malignancy. Although most urologists argue that the small risk inherent in extra testing is far outweighed by the benefits of finding all those extra cancers at a still treatable stage, the number crunchers don't agree. A 1996 review of PSA screening in the *Journal of the American Medical Association* concluded that as it currently stands, PSA screening is reminiscent of screening for lung cancer with X rays—the benefits are still unproven, and perhaps most troubling, the risks may outweigh the benefits.

So that's how the debate currently stands. Urologists just about uniformly believe that all men at average risk for prostate cancer should be screened with regular PSA tests from the age of fifty on, while many epidemiologists, as well as many paying agencies, still believe that PSA screening in low-risk men is not worth the price.

In view of this controversy, whether or not you get a PSA test depends largely on how neurotic you are. The more you worry about such things, the more likely you are to say, "Who cares, anyway? I'll risk the consequences of a false positive test and get my PSA done. Gulp!" Which is exactly what I have done. As a world-class neurotic, I'm afraid I had no choice, and I figure that most men I know would probably do the same, especially since a recent study from Canada concluded that PSA screening could decrease the death rate from prostate cancer by up to 69 per cent. I really want to be in that number.

If you decide to get PSA screening, how often should you have it done? Some pro-PSA experts advise having a yearly test, but a study in the *Journal of Urology* found that in a male with a PSA level below 2.0 ng/ml, every two years is probably enough.

The bitter debate about PSA may, however, soon be put to bed because happily, preliminary research has indicated that free or unbound PSA is a better measure of prostate cancer than total PSA; the test for free PSA seems to be associated with fewer false positives and false negatives than is total PSA. What seems likely to happen soon is that men will be screened for PSA, and when the PSA level is raised, they will then be tested for free PSA. This procedure should make a significant dent in the number of men who are misdirected to ultrasound and biopsy from a falsely high PSA test.

A final point. An interesting study has linked higher blood levels of the hormone insulinlike growth factor-1 (or, more mercifully, IGF-1) with an up to four times higher risk of prostate cancer. This is a preliminary report and must be repeated, but if confirmed, it may give us another tool to help identify men at higher risk.

Treatment   This issue is too complex to tackle here, but I will tell you that there is a lot of controversy about whether it even pays to treat certain prostate cancers. Some evidence suggests that in elderly gents with small tumours, doing nothing, the age-old therapy known as "watchful waiting," is as effective as treatment that is available now. A well-publicized study from Scandinavia found, for example, that elderly men who received the then current best therapy lived an average of sixteen years after diagnosis of prostate cancer; men who elected no therapy also lived an average of about sixteen years after diagnosis. Another study from Denmark found that over one-third of men with localized prostate cancer—cancer that has not spread—will "neither suffer nor die from their disease." The flip side, however, is that two-thirds will die from their disease, most within ten years.

For younger men with prostate cancer, however, the experts agree that something must be done. The problem is deciding what that "something" should be. The factors that you must take into account include the stage of the tumour (a measure of how far the cancer has spread from its nub in the prostate), which is then correlated with a probable prognosis for that kind of cancer; your state of health; the state of the art in your locale (this may get me kicked out of the next physicians' golf tournament held in my area, which would not be that much of a loss, to be sure, since they never invite me anyway, but some doctors and institutions are simply more adept at these procedures than others); what your doctor pushes you to do; and what your life will be like after whatever choice you make (will incontinence, for example, make your life simply unbearable?). The choices are watchful waiting (as noted above), radiation therapy, cryotherapy (freezing of the cells), surgery, and for advanced cancers, hormonal therapy, which includes, alas, a procedure to eliminate sex hormones very like the one that was done on my husky Big Louie at a rather tender age and that has turned him into the largest, most sedate, highest-pitched-howling male Malamute on the continent. Each of these options carries its own risks and benefits.

Surgery is still the standard therapy for most prostate cancers in most of the developed world, an operation that unfortunately may carry some nasty surprises; it can leave you with those twin devils of incontinence and impotence as friends for life. The reason for these complications is simple: the nerves and muscles that are involved in both bladder control and erectile ability are in intimate contact with the prostate and are often unavoidably injured in prostate surgery. The good news, however, is that an American company has just marketed a machine that it claims can help the surgeon avoid slicing the vital nerves involved in maintaining potency. This machine works on the same principle as a metal detector—the closer the machine gets to a nerve, the louder it beeps. Not only that, a really skilled surgeon is also able to find many of the coins that you have lost over your lifetime, although he may have trouble extracting the larger ones.

Radiation therapy used to be reserved only for inoperable tumours or for men who were too weak or too ill to withstand surgery. But a newer technique (called brachytherapy) that employs seeds or pellets of radioactive material that are left in place in the tumour confines most of the effects of radiation to prostate tissue only and carries less risk than older forms of radiation. As a result, radiotherapists are now actively pushing radiotherapy, especially for smaller, localized tumours, although a recent study from some Johns Hopkins investigators has questioned whether radiotherapy works as well as had been hoped even for these select tumours.

Among the newer and more intriguing therapies is vaccine therapy. Researchers in Seattle are conducting advanced vaccine trials on a group of men who have either metastatic prostate cancer or evidence (via a raised PSA) that their prostate cancer has recurred. These researchers take immune cells called dendrites from the cancer patient's blood, multiply those cells in the lab, expose the dendrites to a component of prostate cancer cells so that the altered dendrites can now recognize cancer cells, and reinject these new and wise dendrites back into the patient, where they "teach" other immune cells how to seek and destroy the cancer cells. Strictly speaking, this is not a "vaccine," since its purpose is to combat an already existing disease. But the principle in this trial is the same as in a vaccine.

In another intriguing experiment, using lab mice, researchers from Johns Hopkins University have manipulated a prostate cancer gene, grafted it onto the back of a cold virus, and reinjected it back into the mice, where the virus homed in on the prostate cancer and zapped it.

So there is hope on the horizon, guys. Get yourself a good pair of binoculars and try to hold on until one of those ships comes in.

CHAPTER 5

Dispelling Myths about Disease in Middle Age

Don't it always seem to go
that you don't know what you got till it's gone.

—JONI MITCHELL, "Big Yellow Taxi"

Earlier I sprung the surprising fact on you that most middle-aged men are the original happy gang, the most smug, most self-sufficient, and most self-congratulatory demographic group. There is an important exception to this orgy of self-delusion, however—namely, that cohort of middle-aged guys dealing with chronic illnesses. As my mom is wont to point out, "If you have your health, Arthur, you have everything," and I would take her word on this one, guys, since at last count, my mom did indeed seem to have everything. And she's holding on to it very tightly too.

Happiness, alas, often does largely depend on one's state of health, and sadly, middle age is when a still small but growing number of men start dealing with physical or mental chronic illness, which not only affects their well-being but also limits their life expectancy. To quote from a study in the *British Medical Journal*, "healthy life expectancy is determined by a relatively limited number of chronic conditions that become more common with increasing age." To be fair, the authors of this study were talking about elderly people dealing with problems such as heart disease, osteoporosis, hip fractures, diabetes, strokes, arthritis, neurodegenerative disorders such as memory loss and dementia, cancers, depression, visual loss, cataracts, glaucoma, deafness, and a host of equally cheery conditions. But the first signs of many of these illnesses sprout, like many of our parts, in middle age.

Most of us plan for an old age of contentment, sitting by a fireplace, regaling our mates with tales from our youth. This is an illusion. Although we never plan on getting sick, most of us will.

What follows is a description of some of the diseases that you might run into or that might be worrying you as you wade ever deeper into middle age. This is not meant to be an all-inclusive list. My purpose is to dispel some myths, to alleviate anxiety, to poke fun, to add a pearl of wisdom your other oyster, your family doc, may have missed, to offer my take on controversial aspects of some health issues, and most of all, to push prevention.

Alzheimer's Disease

The only reason I mention Alzheimer's disease is that most baby boomers are terrified that a single instance of misplacing the keys is the first hint of impending Alzheimer's. This is nonsense. A good definition I once heard of Alzheimer's is that although we all forget our keys occasionally, people with Alzheimer's forget what the keys are for. Yes, Alzheimer's is an eventual threat to your health, but with the exception of certain kinds of genetically linked Alzheimer's, not in your middle years. By the time it becomes a real threat to us middle-agers, one hopes that better treatments may be available.

Until that day comes, however, the best bet is to protect yourself with the few preventive measures that scientists believe may make a difference. Thus, a study from Columbia University published in the *Journal of the American Medical Association* concluded that using your brain is important. In this study, people with fewer than eight years of school or those with less-skilled jobs (such as, I suppose, talk show hosts and men who work in city-planning departments) had double the risk of those who had a more advanced education or higher-skilled jobs. So if you do nothing else, get yourself a good education. If you don't already have an advanced degree, however, I doubt that buying one now from one of those mail-order universities will do the trick.

This study also found that once Alzheimer's set in, its course was not affected by level of education. According to the researchers, it's more likely that the more you use your brain in your younger years, the more synapses you develop and the larger the effective "usable" brain area you end up with. And a larger brain gives you more of a cushion against the inevitable deterioration of age.

Regular strenuous exercise throughout life also seems to offer some protection against Alzheimer's. So if you want to keep sharp, run to your adult education courses. In addition, an intriguing recent study claims that a diet high in folic acid may lower the risk of Alzheimer's.

A few studies have linked the regular use of anti-inflammatory drugs to a lower risk of Alzheimer's. Scientists do not know how these drugs work, however, or even if they really work at all. For this reason, until more is known about this potential link, don't start using these potent drugs without consulting your doctor first (see Chapter 8).

You may also have read that estrogen-replacement therapy can lower the risk of Alzheimer's. For most men, however, the side effects of estrogen therapy (bigger breasts, an urge to talk endlessly on the phone) probably outweigh the benefits.

Among the proscriptions occasionally offered to minimize the risks of Alzheimer's are these "don'ts": don't cook with aluminum pots, don't use antiperspirants, don't take antacids, don't brush your teeth with toothpaste, don't drink the water in many parts of the world. All of the foregoing items have been proposed as sources of excess aluminum, a potential toxin to the brain, although I think it's much more likely that Alzheimer's is due to normal changes as a result of aging and to poor lifestyle habits than to the amount of antacid you swallow.

There is one other important "don't" that I want to add to that list. Don't get tested. Alzheimer's has been linked to a higher blood level of a fatty substance called apolipoprotein E, and a test for the presence of this chemical is now available. But if your blood levels are normal, you cannot be assured that you won't eventually get Alzheimer's anyway. If the test is positive, even though this is not a guarantee that you will get Alzheimer's, each time you forget your wife's name, you will be immobilized with fear that this is the first sign of your inevitable decline. Until therapies and preventive strategies that work are available, there is absolutely no reason to get tested for Alzheimer's in middle age.

BACK PAIN

Eighty per cent of adults have experienced at least one episode of acute back pain by the time they hit fifty.

Happily for most of us, acute back pain is a one-off event that responds equally well to any intervention we choose, mainly because the most important aspect of any treatment is tincture of time.

For those guys who simply cannot wait and who require—or more accurately, desire—more than a passing pat on the back when they're hurting and the "You're all right, dear" reassurance that all of our women friends are so quick to offer us when we're in indescribably severe pain, the best thing is to take a few mild analgesics and return to normal activity as soon as possible. What you should not do is lie in bed and feel sorry for yourself. It's not the feeling sorry for yourself that's a concern—it's the bed rest. While lying around and doing nothing for weeks on end may give you something in common with your teenage son, it not only does your back no good but often even allows the pain to linger, since the muscles and other soft tissues, like your son, quickly get used to doing nothing and signal their resentment when even normal activities are reintroduced by sending out painful signals.

As to more active therapies, most studies conclude that it doesn't matter which intervention you choose—chiropractic manipulation, physiotherapy, massage, eating cheese—because they all offer equal relief. Thus, a survey from the University of North Carolina concluded that family doctors, chiropractors, and orthopedic surgeons were all equally good at getting rid of low back pain. Overall, however, patients were most satisfied with chiropractors because they were better at explaining to the patient what was wrong. If you're a Type A like me, however, who hates waiting even a minute for some self-satisfied professional to give you a crumb of his time, most of that chiropractic satisfaction would be offset by the fact that chiropractors demand way more return visits than do the other back-pain specialists.

"I can buy getting back to work quickly, Art," I can hear some of you whining, "and I can even buy not getting therapy. But what I find hard to accept is that you don't suggest any tests—X rays or CT scans—to tell me that I don't have a ruptured disk that might paralyze me in an instant." Sorry, Jack, you just don't need them, because very few cases of acute back pain require investigation. You see, lots of us develop one or more bulging disks in our spinal column as we get older, but these bulging disks, like a bulging waistline, are usually incidental to aging and seldom the cause of our pain. If a surgeon sees one of those incidental bulging discs, however, he may be very tempted to go in and fix it. An old joke: One surgeon says to another, "What did the patient have?" "$800." "No. I mean what did you operate for?" "I told you. $800."

Having said that, you should see your physician immediately if you develop

- sudden sharp back pain that is accompanied by weakness in any part of your lower limbs, especially in your feet or ankles
- pain that is accompanied by any difficulty with urination or bowel movements
- pain that is severe and unrelenting, especially if it is getting worse
- sharp back pain that is accompanied by fever and chills (not chills from the natural fear all men have of even minor pain but chills as a sign of infection)

Finally, a word on prevention. Acute back pain is preventable, if you follow some simple rules your mom told you:

- Keep your weight down.
- Don't smoke (smokers have more back pain than nonsmokers).
- When you have to lift boxes or furniture—as when your wife decides to redesign the living room for the second time that week—bend properly and lift only from the knees.
- Most important, keep in shape.

As to the type of surface to sleep on, opinions differ about which mattress is best, but I figure it's not the type of mattress you sleep on as much as the type of partner you choose to sleep with that matters most.

DEPRESSION

It is generally agreed that about 15 per cent of adults suffer from depression at some point in their lives. Who gets depressed and why? That's easy: anyone can get depressed, and scientists have no idea why. They do know that depression involves changes in brain chemistry, most notably changes in the neurotransmitter serotonin. They also know that certain factors are linked to a higher risk of depression:

- Anyone who has been depressed before is much more likely to become depressed than someone who has not been depressed before.

- A family history of depression is associated with a higher risk of depression.
- Depression is a feature of some metabolic illnesses.
- Several medications, such as calcium channel blockers, the statins for lowering cholesterol, amphetamines, and anabolic steroids can produce depression or at least highlight a latent depression in some people.
- Sleep disturbances are also related to a higher risk of depression. An American study published in the *American Journal of Epidemiology* found that male medical students who had trouble sleeping were twice as likely to be depressed thirty years later as their peers who had no trouble falling asleep.

What may surprise you is that depression has consequences for the rest of your well-being.

- A twenty-seven-year Scandinavian study found that men with "high depressive scores" had an increased risk of death from all causes and a 59 per cent greater risk of heart attack than normal men.
- Middle-aged men with high anxiety levels or depression scores are twice as likely as calm or happy men to develop high blood pressure, with all its attendant health risks, later in life.
- Depressed heart patients hospitalized with chest pains are three times as likely to die over the subsequent year as similar but non-depressed cardiac patients.
- The risk of stroke in men who are depressed is 50 per cent greater than in men who are not depressed.

Symptoms
So there's no getting away from it: depression is linked to many other health risks. That's why it's imperative to recognize depression and to do something about it. But how do you recognize depression? First, you must differentiate depression from a bad mood. Every one of us has occasional bad moods, or so I've heard, that last from a few minutes to days at a time. But depression is much more than that. A major review of depression summarized the more common symptoms as:

- a depressed or irritable mood most of the day, nearly every day
- a diminished interest or pleasure in most activities

- significant weight loss or gain
- insomnia or sleeping too much nearly every day
- agitation or sluggishness most of the time
- fatigue or loss of energy most of the time
- intense feelings of worthlessness
- a drop in ability to concentrate, or indecisiveness
- recurrent thoughts of death or suicide

To this list, you can add features such as loss of appetite and sex drive, and an inability to experience pleasure, although the latter is also present in every member of Generation X, and they couldn't all be depressed, could they? Some depressives also exhibit a heightened level of anxiety, with symptoms such as palpitations, sweating, agitation, phobias, fears, and worries—in short, all the signs a Jewish mother exhibits when her thirty-year-old son is two minutes late coming home. On Saturday afternoon. From synagogue.

Unfortunately, the signs and symptoms of depression are often subtle. Consequently, depression often goes unnoticed for a long time, even years. One survey found, for example, that only one in four depressed people has received therapy. And even when depression is recognized, it is often treated inadequately. According to an expert American panel, fewer than one-third of depressed patients who are given antidepressants take a high enough dose to get their full benefits.

The reason for this poor track record starts with the patient. Many depressed people, the panel concludes, worry about the effects a diagnosis of depression might have either on their job or on their rights to both health and life insurance, so they don't admit their symptoms to a health professional. Some people don't think their symptoms need treatment, or they have come to believe that their sad and negative feelings are normal.

The panel has some harsh words for doctors as well. Many doctors, it seems, spend too little time with patients to pick up the often subtle symptoms of depression, and even when they do diagnose it, they are often too busy to deal with it properly.

Treatment

The best treatment for depression is to prevent it in the first place. Thus, a higher intake of fish, fruits, and veggies has been linked to a lower incidence of depression. But before you rush out to buy up your corner store's supply of eggplant and canned herring, be aware that this diet-depression link may only be a reflection of the fact that people who eat better are less at risk for depression to begin with. Regular exercise has also been promoted as a way to lower one's risk of depression, although a large American study on doctors—perhaps not the most typical group to look at for general principles to apply to the rest of society—failed to find that exercise prevented depression at all.

When it comes to active treatment, the world is divided into talkers and takers. Talkers believe that depression should always be treated with psychotherapy. A taker like me, however, will prefer to get his cure from the insides of a capsule rather than the insights of a fat fool.

The drug du jour, mainly because most people don't think of it as a drug, is St.-John's-Wort. In a widely reported study in Europe, where this herb has been used for over two hundred years, St.-John's-Wort was found to be as effective as synthetic antidepressants for mild to moderate depression.

There is a slew of synthetic antidepressants to choose from, although the newer ssri's (selective serotonin re-uptake inhibitors) have replaced the older tricyclics as drugs of first choice. ssri's boost levels of serotonin in the brain by allowing it to circulate longer. The reason that ssri's have become the favourite drugs for treating depression is threefold: they work; they are more easily tolerated than the older medications, most of which were tricyclic antidepressants; and they also appear to be safer than the tricyclics, especially, perhaps, for heart patients.

The most significant side effects of ssri's are sleep disturbance and sexual dysfunction, such as decreased libido and "delayed orgasm," and the latter is often not a minor problem. For example, a Dutch study found that antidepressant drugs (Luvox was an exception) can "seriously" delay male orgasm. Specifically, time to orgasm (that's two nouns, by the way, not a noun and a verb) was delayed up to eight times longer, long enough, say the researchers, to "disrupt" intercourse, although I figure that most women would be only too happy to have intercourse "disrupted" to eight times its normal length, because that way total time from "What about it?" to "Good night, then" might actually approach several minutes. When you discontinue your medication, you may suffer withdrawal effects such as nausea, dizziness, tremor, anxiety, and palpitations, although these symptoms can often be minimized by gradually tapering the dose.

You should also know that antidepressants don't kick in for at least several days and may take up to several weeks to prove effective. And once you decide to take them, you should continue taking them long enough to let them do all they are meant to do, a period of about six to nine months on the first go-round. If you have been diagnosed with recurring depression, most experts now believe that you should stay on antidepressants for life. There is no reason, however, that you should not try a holiday from drugs whenever you think the time is propitious, after consultation with your doctor. Or better yet, just switch to a placebo. Many studies have found that placebos are also quite effective antidepressants.

Among the myriad other therapies that have also been touted for depression are cognitive behaviour therapy; sleep-deprivation therapy—that is, not being allowed to sleep, thus presumably resetting the biological clock and the brain's neurotransmitters (although I have always wondered, if sleep deprivation is so good at preventing depression, why is postpartum depression often so difficult to deal with?); dance therapy (although its effectiveness probably depends on who your dance partner happens to be); narrative therapy or telling your story (a potential complication here is that your story might depress the hell out of anyone forced to listen to you); acupuncture; art therapy; writing therapy; music therapy; rolfing; this book; and a host of other treatments.

DIABETES

Today diabetes is said to affect 5 to 7 per cent of the population, a sixfold increase since 1958, and this percentage is expected to rise dramatically as more of us baby boomers waddle into middle age. According to a recent American survey, diabetes is now being diagnosed in baby boomers in much higher numbers and often up to two decades earlier than in our parents. Currently, diabetes accounts for one in seven dollars spent on health care. So just imagine how much higher your taxes for health care expenditures are soon going to be thanks to your fellow bulging boomers.

Diabetes is a complex disorder of carbohydrate and protein metabolism manifested in an abnormally high blood glucose (sugar) level, which results in damage to both large and small arteries. There are two types of diabetes, cunningly named Type I diabetes and Type II diabetes. In Type I diabetes, which accounts for 5 to 10 per cent of all diabetes cases, pancreas cells are destroyed, nearly always early in life—hence the old name of juvenile-onset diabetes—resulting in an absolute drop in insulin levels.

Type II diabetes is the animal I want to discuss. It accounts for about 90 per cent of all diabetes cases, and it appeals to my lecturing heart because Type II diabetes is to a huge extent the offspring of an inappropriate lifestyle that eventually causes the body to become "resistant" to insulin. In Type II diabetes, there is usually enough insulin hanging around and trying to do its thing, but for reasons that are still not fully understood, the body is unable to respond normally to this insulin.

The most prevalent theory about why we are witnessing an epidemic of Type II diabetes is that human beings have simply outstripped evolution, a theory that, I admit, flies in the face of such strong empirical counterevidence as Howard Stern, Slobodan Milosevic, curling, infomercials, wwf wrestling, and tv fitness shows. This theory postulates that our ancestors lived in a feast-or-famine state. When they managed to down a mastodon or a sabre-toothed tiger, they gorged on the carcass (at least our carnivore ancestors did; the ones who preferred veggies probably never made it up the evolutionary ladder), and their bodies learned to burn the calories quickly and store what wasn't needed right away as fat, since they could not predict when the next feast or even the next meal would be served up. We, however, are privileged to feast every day, and in the case of my son Tim, several times a day, and our metabolic processes have simply not kept up. Thus, although we don't need all the extra fat those supplemental calories give us, we store the fat anyway, leading to the metabolic changes of Type II diabetes.

Risk factors for Type II diabetes include:

- being overweight
- following a calorie-rich, high-fat diet
- getting older
- living a sedentary life (one study has shown that any exercise at all lowers the risk of developing Type II diabetes)
- having had a previous blood test showing impaired glucose tolerance
- having a parent with Type II diabetes

Excess weight is particularly important. In fact, weight plays such a strong role in Type II diabetes that according to one study, you can reduce your risk with a weight loss as modest as five to ten pounds.

Clearly, however, not everyone is at equal risk of developing Type II diabetes from weight gain alone. After all, we all know some very heavy folks who never develop diabetes. These folks are genetically protected, probably because God didn't want to punish them more than She already had, but you and I, Jocko, are usually not that lucky. God is quite happy to punish us, and diabetes seems to be one of Her preferred ways.

"Big deal," you say. "I'll eat as much as I want and I'll sit on the couch while you do your stupid aerobics, and even if I get diabetes, I'll just take some pills and that's that." But diabetes is not just that. Diabetes is related to a higher risk of stroke, heart attack, blindness, amputation (especially of the feet), kidney failure, and perhaps even dementia. Diabetes also produces nerve damage; signs of nerve damage will develop in nearly half those people who have Type II diabetes within ten years of their being diagnosed. This is a disease worth preventing.

It's easy to diagnose Type II diabetes in someone who starts drinking huge amounts of water, who runs to the bathroom several extra times a day (and night), and who is also feeling very tired and losing weight. But the experts claim that 50 per cent of people with Type II diabetes don't know they have it (the average patient is said to have had diabetes for six years before it was diagnosed), because in the early stages the symptoms can be quite subtle. So since symptoms are not an adequate gauge, it just makes sense for middle-aged men to have regular blood sugar tests. A reading over 126 mg/dL (6.9 nmol/L) is considered abnormal.

If you have already developed Type II diabetes, to control your blood sugar levels:

- You must, you must, you must get down as close to your desirable weight as you can get (and I don't mean the weight you desire to get to, which is probably thirty pounds too much, but the weight the charts tell you is the most desirable for your height).
- You must start doing exercise.
- You must moderate your consumption of alcohol.
- You must limit your intake of high-calorie, high-fat foods.

In addition, an American study has shown that intravenous vitamin C helped control blood sugar levels in diabetics. I do not advise you to start shooting up vitamin C pills, but a diet high in antioxidant-rich fruits and vegetables might help.

It's also very important to have frequent blood tests to help you gauge how well you are controlling your blood sugar levels. I don't mean just those blood glucose tests you can do on your own at home—you must also have regular, more specialized tests that monitor how well you're controlling your blood sugar over the long term. Several medications help control blood sugar, and researchers are also actively pursuing revolutionary new therapies such as transplantation of pancreatic cells, insulin in pill form, and artificial pancreases.

A couple of other notes about treatment: one study found "spectacular" results from using chromium in elderly Chinese with Type II diabetes, so you might want to talk to your doctor about this, especially, I suppose, if you are an elderly Chinese person, and another study found that treating depression in diabetics helps them control their blood sugar levels more easily. So if you're a depressed diabetic, take Hamlet's advice to Ophelia and "get thee to a therapy" ASAP.

GASTROESOPHAGEAL REFLUX DISEASE

In gastroesophageal reflux disease, hydrochloric acid washes back from the stomach into the esophagus. Now as you would expect, the esophagus is no different from you and me. It too doesn't enjoy getting burned by acid, and eventually the washed-up acid irritates the esophagus enough to produce esophagitis, or inflammation of the esophagus. Most people with esophagitis are able to control it with appropriate therapy, but in about a quarter of cases the esophagitis becomes recurrent, persistent, and progressive, and eventually the irritated and altered esophageal lining can develop premalignant changes. Chew on that news for a while as you swallow another antacid, or three.

A quick word about hiatus hernia. A hiatus hernia occurs when the diaphragm weakens. The diaphragm is the muscle that separates the thoracic cavity, which contains the lungs and heart, from the abdominal cavity, which contains the stomach and bowels and other bits. There is a tight opening in the diaphragm through which the esophagus slides into the stomach, and when that tight opening widens, parts

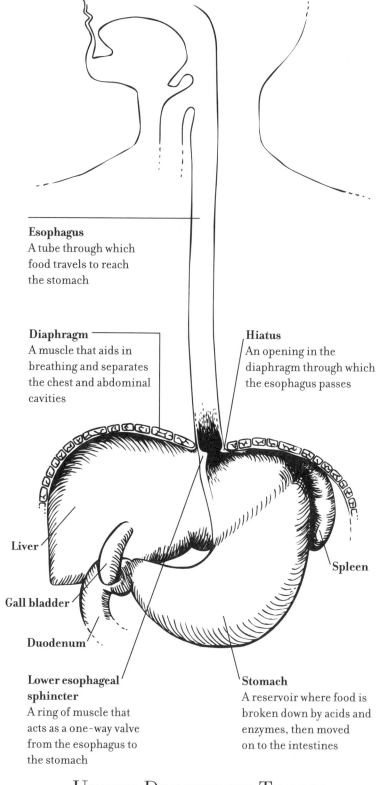

Esophagus
A tube through which
food travels to reach
the stomach

Diaphragm
A muscle that aids in
breathing and separates
the chest and abdominal
cavities

Hiatus
An opening in the
diaphragm through which
the esophagus passes

Liver

Spleen

Gall bladder

Duodenum

**Lower esophageal
sphincter**
A ring of muscle that
acts as a one-way valve
from the esophagus to
the stomach

Stomach
A reservoir where food is
broken down by acids and
enzymes, then moved
on to the intestines

UPPER DIGESTIVE TRACT

Adapted from *Gastroesophageal Reflux Disease: A Look at Medical Treatment
and Laparoscopic Surgery.* © 1995 by Krames Communications.

of the stomach can slide upwards, creating a hiatus hernia. A hiatus hernia can be silent, and it can also be associated with reflux, but just because you are diagnosed with a hiatus hernia does not necessarily mean you have reflux disease too.

Gastroesophageal reflux is extremely common. Thirty per cent of adults experience symptoms frequently, and 10 per cent of us have daily symptoms. The symptoms most commonly associated with reflux are:

- regurgitation of stomach contents into the mouth
- heartburn, which is really any burning sensation from just north of the belly button to the back of the throat

Reflux disease can also rear its ugly head by producing

- chest pain,
- hoarseness, especially in the morning (after you have been lying down for several hours and the acid has had a field night inflaming your throat),
- a persistent sore throat,
- and the symptom that I particularly want to flag—coughing or wheezing, especially at night. Nocturnal asthma is often caused by the washing up of acid to irritate the lungs when you lie down, and asthmatics who wake up wheezing and hacking and feeling short of breath should consider their stomachs a possible source of the problem.

Gastroesophageal reflux disease is most accurately diagnosed not by an expert you saw on *Oprah* but by investigations that involve a look down the gullet and into the stomach. If this kind of validation were required for every case, however, gastroenterologists would be so busy looking down the bow that they would have no time left for the stern, an end many of these guys actually prefer for reasons I refuse to speculate about. Thus, most suspected cases of gastroesophageal reflux disease in middle age can and should be treated with a trial of therapy, and only when this fails or when the condition is persistent or progressive does the syndrome require investigation.

You can take the following steps to improve reflux:

- Lose some weight. Yup, that again. The more you weigh, the worse your symptoms.
- Wait several hours after a meal before lying down.
- Avoid straining (even bending over) and exercising after eating.
- Do not wear a tight belt (or if you do, wear it plumber-belly fashion down around your knees).
- Don't smoke.
- Elevate the head of your bed. Some experts advise putting phone books under the head of the bed, although if your reflux is as bad as mine, you probably won't get relief even if you sleep standing up.

As to dietary changes, it's the usual whole enchilada. Actually, an enchilada might not be a good idea, since fatty foods put a strain on the esophageal-stomach barrier and make reflux worse. Go easy on alcohol and caffeine, avoid foods that worsen your symptoms, such as chocolate or onions, don't eat within at least two hours of going to bed, and try to eat small, more frequent meals rather than one or two large ones.

Most people with gastroesophageal reflux disease self-medicate with antacids or the newer acid-suppressing drugs that are now available over the counter. These drugs work well in mild cases. You should never, however, self-medicate for more than a few weeks without discussing your symptoms with a physician. When you have to move beyond self-medication, there are a host of drugs to choose from, but the ones fast becoming most popular are proton pump inhibitors such as omeprazole, which are very effective. The usual caveat applies, however: the complete safety of these drugs over the long term has not been established, so be cautious about this kind of long-term commitment. Happily, avoiding a long-term commitment is something that many men find relatively easy to do.

Remember also that if you have to take any of these drugs for chronic persistent esophagitis, you need to have your esophagus checked regularly.

HEART DISEASE

Heart disease is the number one killer in North America. In fact, the lethal combo of heart disease and stroke, a disease with nearly all the same roots as heart disease, is responsible for nearly half of all deaths in North American men. So the more familiar you become with this duo, the greater the chances that you might do something about these often silent killers, and the longer you might be around to buy the next book I am working on: *Men in Slippers, or Geezers: The Shuffling of North America*.

To understand heart disease, you need to know about arteries and what damages them. Atherosclerotic disease refers to the narrowing of arteries due to the buildup of fatty substances, calcium, and clotting material on the inside of any artery wall. The accumulation of this arterial crud and garbage in the coronary arteries, the arteries that supply blood to the heart, is called coronary heart disease. Most heart attacks occur because the plugs (or plaques) that build up in the coronary arteries split and cause a clot to develop, which prevents blood from reaching parts of the heart tissue. The symptoms of a heart attack are:

- chest pain that is usually described as crushing or vicelike (although it is often much more subtle) and that can radiate to the jaw, neck, left arm, or back
- sweating
- anxiety
- nausea
- shortness of breath, also known as SOB (curiously, SOB also often describes the guy who's just had a heart attack, and many times his doctor as well)

Atherosclerotic disease is also the leading cause of heart failure and stroke, what some experts have begun to call a brain attack, when the blood vessels to the brain plug up. According to a Dutch study, atherosclerotic disease can also cause a great deal of cognitive impairment that is not just related to age. The researchers claim that the subjects of their study would have had much better cognitive abilities if they had not at the same time been suffering from atherosclerosis.

Risk Factors
Factors related to a higher risk of heart disease include:

- smoking
- a strong family history of premature heart disease or stroke (generally defined as a first-degree relative who was diagnosed with heart disease or a stroke before the age of fifty-five)

- high cholesterol levels
- high blood pressure
- excessive alcohol intake
- diabetes
- obesity
- being too sedentary
- excess stress

I have already discussed diabetes, and I will discuss obesity and alcohol in Chapters 6 and 7. I will also assume that you are smart enough to know that smoking greatly increases your risk of heart disease, and that you don't need any lectures from me to convince you to stop smoking if you want to save your heart.

I do, however, want to take some space talking about three important risk factors: high cholesterol levels, high blood pressure, and stress.

Cholesterol Levels   Lipids are fats (my kids have nicknamed me Lipid, by the way). Lipoproteins are compounds of fatty substances and proteins that serve as a transport system to deliver fats to your tissues. Most cholesterol, a type of fat, is carried in the bloodstream as part of low-density lipoproteins (LDL), the so-called bad cholesterol. When LDL is oxidized and deposited into the walls of already damaged arteries, it plugs those arteries even further. Some cholesterol is carried as high-density lipoproteins (HDL), the so-called good cholesterol, and for reasons that are still not well understood, high HDL levels somehow protect your arteries and inhibit some of the damage LDL can do. Triglycerides are fats carried in the blood on the backs of very-low-density lipoproteins (VLDL). In a still-imperfectly understood manner, triglycerides can be bad for damaged arteries as well.

Now I realize that what you have just read is a real plateful, so if you're getting overwhelmed, just remember this: High HDL = Good. High LDL = Bad. High VLDL = Bad. You got that? Good boy. You don't really need much more background information, so just hang in there. The more saturated fats you take in, the higher your risk of heart attack, both in the short term and in the long term. In the short term, eating a high-fat meal raises the concentration of a clotting factor in the blood and thus raises your immediate risk of a heart attack for several hours following the meal. Thus, after you gorge on a typical yuppie meal of pork bellies and brie, you should try to remain in hailing distance of a cardiac ward.

In the long term—and it's actually the long term that gets most men—the more bacon and steak fat and cream cheese and other saturated fats you send down your gullet, the more the LDL and VLDL transports steam into your already narrowed arteries to deposit their thick goo and sludge and plug those narrow channels even more. Think of those cruise ships that visit Skagway or Vera Cruz and unload their tons of tubby tourists, who immediately plug up the narrowed streets of the town they take over.

So here's one more equation to remember. Saturated fats = BAD, BAD, BAD. What were the other equations, by the way? No peeking.

As with love and a car rental charge, however, there is more to these fats equations than first meets the eye. For example, there are genetic and enzyme differences in how we handle our fatty loads. Thus, some men unload those LDL and VLDL cargo ships much more swiftly and disperse their dangerous cargo more efficiently than do other men.

Unfortunately, doctors still haven't figured out all the genes and enzymes involved in this transport system, so for now, probably the best way to judge how high your risk is from this lipid convoy is through your full blood cholesterol profile. Generally, you want

- your total cholesterol level to be below 5.2 mmol/L (200 mg/dL)
- your LDL level to be below 3.6 mmol/L (130 mg/dL)
- your HDL level to be above .90 mmol/L (35 mg/dL)
- your triglyceride level to be below 2.29 mmol/L (200 mg/dL)
- your VLDL to be below 1.0 mmol/L (39 mg/dL)

I can't tell you how many men call my radio show and whine, "Hey, Doc! My cholesterol level is getting quite high. What should I do?" Sell, of course. I mean this is like asking someone, "If I tell you the name of one character in a play, can you tell me if the play will be any good?" If you are going to get your cholesterol levels checked, as I think every one of you should at least once by middle age (and to hell with what the number-crunching health authorities think about the cost; if they're so keen to save tax and health care dollars, let them work for free), always ask for a full cholesterol profile. And be sure to remember the numbers.

These are only general guidelines, however, and other factors must be considered along with cholesterol levels in evaluating the risk from those levels. Or to quote the wise words of an old free clinic hippie patient of mine whose name was Doc (I don't think he was an MD, although he was certainly a specialist in smoking), "Hey, dude! One man's high is just another man's mellow." Thus, a man with a history of premature death from heart disease in his family probably requires much more attention, and probably more intervention at lower, perhaps even high normal, cholesterol levels, than does a man whose grandparents lived to a ripe old age and whose parents both expired in their nineties while making love for the third time that day.

Happily, most of us can improve our cholesterol levels somewhat through appropriate lifestyle changes. So let's agree that whether your cholesterol levels are "high" or not, but especially if they are:

- You will stop smoking.
- You will do more exercise.
- You will try to get your weight down.
- You will try hard as hell to reduce your stress level.

As part of that stress reduction, you might also consider starting to take all those supplements and nutritional aids that your health-nut friends have assured you are bound to save your life and that are reputed to work much better than drugs, stuff like garlic, lecithin, vitamins C and E, and a host of others. One supplement I would advise against, however, is fish oil capsules because these have still not established their worth in independent studies, but even more because fish are very complicated animals, and surely when God put them together, She meant for you to eat the whole carp or pike and not to just extract some fatty juice from its skin and meat. Remember, however, that taking supplements and nutritional aids does not replace the need to make all those other lifestyle adjustments.

You will also investigate how to change your diet, although this is not as easy as it may seem because to a very large extent, our genes determine whether following a low-fat diet is going to help us or not; some men who go on a low-fat diet actually experience a worsening of their lipid levels. Besides, a British study from the University of Sheffield concluded that going on a low-fat diet increases anger and hostility (no kidding!) and may even make some people depressed. A much better plan than simply lowering fat intake is to change your diet to a more

Mediterranean-style cuisine by eating way more fruits, veggies, grains, beans, and fibre; by replacing a lot of your saturated fats with polyunsaturated fats such as sunflower oil and safflower oil and especially mono-unsaturated fats such as olive oil; by decreasing your intake of meat, especially red meat; and by increasing your intake of fish because studies have linked regular fish eating with a better lipid profile, less heart disease, and lower risk of dying from sudden death, which is usually caused by an abnormality in heart rhythm.

Most important, you will work very, very hard at all these adjustments because according to a four-year study from Dr. Dean Ornish, even men with severe heart disease were able to reduce the narrowing in their coronary arteries with a very low-fat diet, stress reduction, and a moderate amount of exercise. You will also make absolutely sure to get your partner onside because the British Family Heart Study found that it's much easier to get people to change their poor health habits if the efforts to change are geared to the couple or family instead of simply to the individual at risk.

After making the aforementioned adjustments, you will get retested several months down the road. If, however, like you, your cholesterol levels also refuse to budge much, you will now talk to your doctor about whether you should be taking ASA regularly (see Chapter 6) and about whether drugs are the most appropriate therapy. If you both agree that drugs are the best way to go (and this is an area in which I urge you to become as knowledgeable as you can because there is still a good deal of disagreement among the experts about how to proceed), you must next decide which cholesterol-lowering drug is best for you.

The most important thing to know about cholesterol-lowering drugs is that not everyone benefits equally, or even at all, from these medications, because again, genes determine just how well people respond to these drugs. That is why your doctor must be knowledgeable about all these drugs and not just the ones that he has in his drawer or the ones he has seen the pretty ads for. And although this may seem like a silly bit of advice, you actually have to take the drugs for them to do you any good. Studies have shown, you see, that lots of people stop taking their cholesterol-lowering medications when the prescription runs out. This is not a one-shot deal. These drugs are not antibiotics— they generally have to be taken for life.

I really can't leave this discussion without commenting on the controversial and relatively consistent finding in many studies that lowering cholesterol levels is accompanied by an increased risk of depression and a consequent increased risk of dying from suicide and homicide. I must admit that I have always been quite partial to this link because I figure that if some doctor tried to make me stick to a low-cholesterol regime for life, I would surely kill her or, if I couldn't get at her, I would kill myself.

On the ever present other hand, most studies have not found a link between violent death and cholesterol-lowering therapy, and clearly, in the majority of men with significantly raised cholesterol levels, the benefits obtained by improving their cholesterol levels outweigh any potential risk of depression. Nonetheless, if you are on cholesterol-lowering medication, you and your physician should be vigilant for signs of depression, and your physician should be especially wary if you start displaying any interest in joining a gun club.

High Blood Pressure   High blood pressure damages your arteries and multiplies your risk of suffering all those negative consequences that abnormal lipid levels lead to.

For most middle-aged men, a desirable blood pressure reading is anything below 140/90. What may surprise you to learn, though, is that it's not as easy to determine your average blood pressure as you might think. For example, in the last few years a phenomenon known as "white coat hypertension" has received much attention. Men who have this condition get an elevated blood pressure only when it's taken by a health professional, especially some hurry-up passive-aggressive physician visibly anxious to get to the twenty-four other much sicker people in his exam rooms. If these guys get their blood pressure taken by a nice mellow machine, however, or better yet, by an attractive member of the sex they prefer, their blood pressure is often normal. What is still not known, however, is whether white coat hypertension needs to be treated. The main lesson from all this, though, is that you should never rely on one abnormal blood pressure reading as an indication for treatment (see below).

Although raised blood pressure can occasionally be secondary to other problems (kidney disease, other metabolic illnesses, such as hyperthyroidism), over 90 per cent of hypertension is not linked to other conditions and has no known cause, although all the usual suspects—excess weight, too much alcohol, genetic factors, smoking, bad diet, and sitting on your behind—contribute to this one too.

Psychological factors also play a role. A study from Cornell University, for example, concluded that the strain of certain modern jobs with high demands but over which the worker has little control cause "millions of cases" of high blood pressure. High levels of anxiety and depression in middle age have also been shown to be flags for the development of high blood pressure in the future. Your personality, or lack of one, is also a factor, in that pessimists have higher blood pressure than do optimists, but then if you're a pessimist, you were probably already expecting that bad news.

Why is high blood pressure dangerous? Because it injures arteries. The higher your blood pressure, the greater your risk of suffering a heart attack, a stroke, kidney failure, dementia, and a host of other debilitating conditions.

Prevention includes all the old standbys, such as:

- watching your weight
- not smoking
- exercising
- keeping your cholesterol levels down
- moderating your alcohol intake
- reducing your stress load (very important)

How much exercise? What kind of stress reduction? "Whatever works for you," is the answer, and to that end, you might be interested to learn that in a study of older adults, tai chi, the ancient low-intensity Chinese physical activity program, was found to reduce blood pressure nearly as much as did moderate-intensity exercise. One of the side effects of tai chi, however, is that an hour after you've finished the exercise session, you're hungry to do it again.

Many studies have linked a diet rich in potassium with lower blood pressure. So eat lots of bananas, raisins, and apricots.

As to salt, the latest consensus seems to be that although most people with high blood pressure probably do not need to restrict their salt intake much, some do, especially the elderly and black Americans. If your blood pressure is normal, however, there is no reason to believe that salting your food to make it more palatable will turn you into a hypertensive.

One high blood pressure reading, like most presidential protestations of innocence or a government announcement of a tax break, is not to be accepted at face value, so if you are told that you have high blood pressure, the first thing to do is demand a recount. Have it rechecked at least two more times when you are as relaxed as possible —even talking can raise your blood pressure. If your blood pressure is high on three or more occasions, and you have shut up while it was being taken, you must then decide if it is high enough and if you have enough other risk factors for coronary heart disease to necessitate a lifelong commitment to medications. For men with minimally elevated blood pressure, this is likely to be a minefield in which you are going to have to call on all the high school algebra you ever learned to help you figure out the real risk/benefit ratio of a particular medication and the best dose to use. Just remember that most of the studies that have shown a benefit from lowering blood pressure involved the use of older—and much cheaper—medications, such as diuretics and beta-blockers.

Taking medications for high blood pressure is often a lifelong commitment, and like other such permanent commitments that end up lasting only a few years, this one needs to be reevaluated every so often. Up to 30 per cent of older people with high blood pressure can gradually withdraw from medication, and hey, if older people can do it, why not younger ones too? Even if you stop taking medication, however, you should continue to get your blood pressure checked regularly.

Stress   Let me get the easy part out of the way quickly—namely, physical stress. An American study that received lots of media attention found that in previously largely sedentary men (and any men who are primarily sedentary are certainly also large), sudden bursts of activity such as mowing the lawn or shovelling snow off the driveway can lead to sudden death from the rupture of a plaque on the walls of a sick coronary artery. What may scare many of you is that this type of sudden death seems to happen mostly to men in their fifties.

So if sudden bursts of heavy exertion can cause a heart attack, that no doubt immediately brings up the question in most men's minds, and their wives' minds too, I'm sure, what about sex? Sex can kill, I'm afraid, but it should not be your major worry. Although sexual intercourse does slightly increase one's risk of a heart attack, the chance that any individual sex act might set off a heart attack has been estimated to be about one in a million (the mind boggles at some findings; I mean, do you think the researchers went up to guys being resuscitated in the emergency room and asked, "Excuse me, sir, but were you having sex just before you keeled over? Sir? Sir?"). And this risk remains higher for about two hours after the sex act. In other words, it's a two-hour, three-minute total risk for most men.

Probably of greater worry to us aging men is that this study also found that 10 per cent of heart attacks are triggered by simply rising from sleep in the morning. And no, I'm afraid that my son's solution of staying in bed until the afternoon is not the way to deal with this finding.

Now for the hard part: mental stress. How bad is mental stress for your heart? Baaaad. Stressful events have been shown to lead to a rise in blood pressure and pulse rate, to cause abnormalities in heart rhythm, to cause platelets (blood cells vital in clotting) to become stickier and thus to clot more easily, and to produce cardiac ischemia, or decreased blood flow to heart tissue. No wonder, then, that acute and chronic stress are both related to a higher risk of heart attack and sudden death. But what has also become clear is that men with pre-existing heart disease as well as men with certain personality types are more at risk from stressful events than other men.

What kind of personality types? That's the hard part. Several decades ago, some American researchers identified having a Type A personality as an important link to a higher risk of heart attacks from stress. A Type A man—the kind of man who is driven and intense, cuts into line, finishes other people's sentences for them, and counts the number of items other shoppers have in their baskets in the express check-out line (you have no idea how many people with too many items have tried to sneak by me, by the way) is much more at risk, these researchers said, of heart attack when compared to his more laid-back Type B brothers. And this Type A–Type B dichotomy was the accepted theory for many years. But over time it became clear that although some Type A men are indeed at much higher risk of calamitous cardiac events, many Type A men do very well. So, in the last few years, the experts have begun to focus on certain attitudes or features of personality, especially of a Type A personality, as being more predictive of an increased risk of heart attack.

They have particularly singled out hostility as an important personality trait linked to a higher risk of having a heart attack. So how do they describe a hostile man, many of you are probably angrily asking your spouse? As a distrustful man who is not only quick to become angry but who is also more likely to act on his anger—a lane-changing horn honker, in other words. Leaving aside the issue that really burns me up—namely, how the hell do these guys have the chutzpah to try to define a great driver like me as a hostile person—there is some evidence, I must admit, although it makes my blood boil to do so, that being hostile may be bad for you. Thus, hostile males were found to have lower HDL and higher LDL levels at age nineteen and to suffer from more "bad habits," such as smoking and excess alcohol intake, at age forty-two than did their more accommodating brothers; hostile men have been found to have higher blood pressure even during their sleep than their more even-tempered incredibly naïve brothers; and Finns with cynical hostility (cynical hostility—now what kind of nebulous crap is that, I ask you?) have an increased risk of death from all causes compared to non-hostile Finns.

Lately, some researchers have proposed a subcategory under hostility—what they call "dominance"—as another character trait worthy of attention. A study from Duke University found that dominant men—guys who always feel compelled to be the centre of what's going on and who interrupt conversations (but how else can you get your important opinions in?)—were 60 per cent more likely to die during the twenty-two-year study than were their less intrusive brothers.

Another aspect of personality that might play a role in a higher risk of heart attack is chronic anxiety. Thus, men who complain of being very anxious are four to six times as likely to die from a sudden heart attack than their more laid-back brothers. A special type of anxiety is manifested by men who suffer from what researchers in one study called "heightened vigilance," or just being constantly tense about the potential dangers in your environment—for example, always watching out for ladders not to walk under, worrying about the effects shampoo can have on your sperm count, or in my case, being constantly on guard for one of my mother's famous double-ended questions (an old joke: a Jewish son comes down to dinner wearing one of the two ties his mother gave him, and she asks, "So, Melvin, what's wrong with the other one?"). Heightened vigilance was shown to produce "heightened cardiovascular reactivity," which can damage heart tissue and raise the risk of sudden death.

To complicate matters, a study from Belgium has proposed that a Type D personality also has a greater risk of dying from coronary heart disease than other personality types. And what the hell is a Type D, you cynically hostile men no doubt want to know. A Type D is a negative, insecure, and distressed man, a guy who worries excessively, lacks assertiveness, and suppresses his "emotional distress," more Woody Allen than Jack Nicholson, in other words. In this study, Type D guys had three times the risk of suffering a heart attack as did non-Type D men. And to make you Type Ds feel even worse, this study also found that Type D traits are much harder to change than are other potentially harmful personality traits. So if you're a Type D, buddy, do you ever have a lot to worry about, although you're probably doing a heap of worrying already anyway.

So what should you do, if you are one of these high-risk guys? First, get a good lawyer, because you're likely to need one eventually. And then work on the way you handle stress. It might just save your life. For example, Dr. Meyer Friedman (one of the men who first described the Type A personality) and co-workers found that modifying certain Type A personality traits in men who had already suffered a heart attack can halve their risk of suffering a second one. But that still begs the question of how you change. There are many things you can do for yourself (see Chapter 7), but if those are not enough, the best way to learn to modify your stress response is to find a stress management program that's right for you. And stress management programs do work. One study has shown that heart disease patients who learn to manage stress through biofeedback and relaxation are over 70 per cent less likely to have a heart attack than patients who receive only standard medical care.

If programs are not for you, you can try pills instead. A recent study found that the ssri antidepressant paroxetine (Paxil) appears to "reduce hostility and may even boost cooperative behavior," although you first have to cooperate enough to take the bloody pill in the first place. Oops! Must be time for another of those pills.

Other Possible Risk Factors   Homocysteine, an amino acid produced from the breakdown of another amino acid, methionine, has recently been identified as a possible risk factor for heart disease. The best way to lower your homocysteine level is to eat more foods containing vitamin B$_6$ and folic acid (and perhaps vitamin B$_{12}$ as well), and that's good advice no matter what role homocysteine may turn out to have or not have in heart disease.

Several studies have found a link between high iron stores in the body and a higher risk of heart attack, and a study from Kansas University Medical Centre found that donating one unit of blood every three years reduced the risk of a heart attack by 30 per cent. So go ahead, man. Give them a pint every so often. Not only will it allow you to act excessively self-righteous, it might even be good for you. And it will certainly help others.

The last few years, a number of experts have proposed an intriguing link between heart attacks and infections. Thus, for example, a study in the journal *Chest* found that heart attacks in younger men may be initiated by an infection with an organism called *Chlamydia pneumoniae*. So don't get infected. Next.

One final word about heart disease and it's probably the most important advice: don't spend too much time worrying about it. Do the best you can and then get on with your life. According to Dr. James Muller of Deaconess Hospital, Harvard Medical School, who was quoted in *USA Today*, "If a person did everything he could to avoid triggering a heart attack, he'd probably die of boredom."

OSTEOARTHRITIS

Rheumatologists recognize over one hundred forms of arthritis (I have no idea how many they can't recognize), but the only one I want to discuss is osteoarthritis, or degenerative arthritis. About 70 per cent of adults over the age of sixty have some degree of osteoarthritis, produced by deterioration in the articular cartilage in a joint, the cartilage that cushions movement between bones. No wonder, then, that the major symptoms of osteoarthritis are pain, stiffness, crackling sounds in the joint, and joint swelling.

The joints most commonly affected by osteoarthritis are the weight-bearing ones, such as the knees and hips, as well as those in the spine and thumbs. Osteoarthritis of the knee is often cited as the leading cause of disability in elderly North Americans, and the risk of getting it goes up directly with weight. A study of physicians found that the heavier a guy is in his younger years (read: now), the greater his eventual risk of osteoarthritis of the hip or knee (read: soon). Other factors that increase the risk of osteoarthritis are a positive family history, injury to the joint, malalignment of the bones, and calcium deposits or other inflammation in or around the joint.

Once again, treatment starts with prevention. So never get injured. You're welcome. What is perhaps more feasible is to avoid excess weight, and if you are already overweight, to lose as many of those excess pounds as you can, although I don't think losing weight is nearly as important if osteoarthritis affects your thumb as when it affects your knee or back. In addition, a recent study claims that elite athletes seem to have a higher risk of degenerative arthritis, but somehow I don't think that's going to matter much to too many of my readers.

Exercise improves physical performance and lessens pain. Also, figure out which activities trigger your pain and how much of each trigger is required for the pain to set in, and then try to adjust your pain-control strategies to minimize the effects of that trigger. So, for example, if your daily three-mile walk always sets off enough pain to require you to take medication afterwards, you might think of taking a nonsteroidal anti-inflammatory or acetaminophen as a prophylactic measure before the exercise. This doesn't mean that you put a condom on when you set out on the walk; it means that you take the pill before starting the activity. This may lessen your need for even more medication afterwards. As to what to eat, a diet high in fish oils has been linked to less joint inflammation, so it's worth a try. After all, a trout a day certainly beats taking tons of Tylenol. In addition, the multi-faceted Framingham Study, which has been charting the health of the citizens of Framingham, Massachusetts, for nearly five decades, has revealed that a diet high in vitamins C and D is linked to a lower risk of osteoarthritis, and even if the disease sets in anyway, a diet high in these two vitamins slows its progression. Higher doses of vitamin E and beta-carotene have no effect, however.

Standard therapies for osteoarthritis have long included some physical treatment, such as physiotherapy, as well as analgesics such as acetaminophen, ASA, and other anti-inflammatory medications, including sometimes even cortisone.

Recently there has been lots of excitement about glucosamine and chondroitin sulfate, two natural substances involved in the formation of cartilage that have long been used in animals and in Europe (no connection there as far as I can tell). Their proponents claim that these two substances can rebuild joint cartilage. Although there is no proof that they actually do that, there is mounting empirical evidence that they do decrease pain and inflammation in joints affected with osteoarthritis.

In lab studies, doxycycline, a member of the tetracycline family, has been shown to block the enzymes involved in cartilage breakdown. Stay tuned.

One thing you shouldn't do for your joint pain, however, is move somewhere with a warmer climate, such as Arizona or California. For years, doctors in Montreal, where I first practised, used to tell their complaining arthritic patients, "Oyy! Morris! If you could just move to Arizona, Morris, you would be so much better. Arizona, Morris. That's where you should move, and believe me, your pain will be gone. A bege-zunt!" Why? Because the doctor knew that even if the move didn't help Morris, at least the doctor's discomfort would improve the instant Morris toted his tush to Tucson. But according to a study in the journal *Pain*, there really is no one best climate for arthritis. Weather, this study found, affects people's perception of pain no matter where they live, so the best thing to do is to sit tight and continue to kvetch at home.

OSTEOPOROSIS

About one-third of all hip fractures occur in men. Twenty per cent of men who break their hips die within a year of the fracture, and 50 per cent never regain their full mobility. Osteoporosis also affects the spine and leads to fractures in the bones of the spinal column, which not only cause a great deal of pain but also produce a consequent loss of height with age, a sobering prospect for a man of five foot six like me, or at least it used to be five foot six.

The risk factors for osteoporosis are the same in men as in women. Men who have the greatest risk of brittle bones and fractures include those who:

- are smokers
- are Caucasian or Asian
- drink excessive amounts of alcohol
- have a strong family history of osteoporosis
- are sedentary
- have too much protein and too little calcium in their diets
- don't get enough vitamin D (vitamin D helps calcium get absorbed)
- are aging
- have low testosterone levels
- have prematurely grey hair (happily, balding is not a risk factor)

Some drugs, such as steroids, thyroid hormone, and anticonvulsants also rob the bones of calcium.

For prevention, the usual applies:

- Consume enough calcium, starting early in life.
- Watch your alcohol intake.
- Don't smoke.
- Do more weight-bearing exercise.

As to how you get enough calcium, you should rely on your diet and not on supplements. High-calcium foods include dairy products, broccoli, tofu, beans, shrimp, sardines, and salmon bones, although you're not going to stick with this diet for very long, I think, if you sit down to a daily evening meal of soy cubes, sardines, salmon bones, and beans, so don't try to stuff yourself with too much calcium at every dinner.

If you just can't ingest the 1000 to 1500 or so mg of daily calcium you're supposed to take in, then you have to turn to calcium supplements. Calcium citrate is less likely to cause stomach upsets than calcium carbonate, but no matter which form you take, you should also be sure to get enough vitamin D by getting some sun exposure (ten minutes a day is probably enough). If you live in a city like Vancouver, however, getting that amount of sunshine is impossible nine months a year, so you might prefer to eat more vitamin D–enriched foods or to take vitamin D supplements. By the way, my mom swears that the easiest and cheapest way to get enough calcium is to take four or five Tums a day, and although I can't comment about the"easiest" part, I bet you she's right about the "cheapest" part. That's one area where that woman has never been wrong.

Periodontal Disease

As opposed to those media stars who have their own personal trainer, I have instead engaged the services of a personal periodontist, a dentist who specializes in gum disease. Why? In part because I couldn't afford a personal trainer (although the bills from my periodontist have been climbing so rapidly that I think he may be supporting his own personal trainer), but mostly because I need the services of a periodontist so much more. Like many people my age, I have developed periodontal disease, a chronic, persistent, and (in my severe case) painful inflammation of the gums and supporting structures of the teeth.

The earliest stage of periodontal disease is gingivitis, an inflammation caused by the buildup of plaque. Depending on its severity, periodontal disease produces such symptoms as bleeding, swollen, red, and tender gums, as well as bad breath and a bad taste in the mouth. If allowed to proceed unchecked, periodontal disease leads to gum recession, loose teeth, and changes in tooth position, which is why periodontal disease has become the most common cause of tooth loss in people over the age of forty. In fact, my periodontist is fond of telling me as I lie back in his chair, captive and rubber-dammed, "You know, your teeth are in great shape, Art. It's your gums that will have to come out. Open wider."

The treatment for periodontal disease is proper dental care, regular flossing and teeth cleaning, and occasionally, taking antibiotics to kill the bacteria. Perhaps the most important aspect of treatment, though, is to try to find a periodontist who is actually funny, although you may in the end be searching for an oxymoron.

STROKE

The only thing I want to say about strokes is that you should familiarize yourself with how to recognize the signs of a stroke, although I sincerely hope you never have to use this information. There is some evidence that quickly treating the most common kind of strokes, the ones caused by blockage in the arterial supply to a part of the brain, can limit some of the damage, much as treating a heart attack within several hours can result in saving much more heart tissue. Unhappily, however, according to a study, more than 50 per cent of people at increased risk for a stroke are unaware of it, and only about 25 per cent of stroke patients correctly identified their symptoms as stroke related —that is, 75 per cent did not.

This is especially important information, then, for those at high risk of stroke, including anyone with atrial fibrillation, high blood pressure, or heart disease, and anyone who has been told that his carotid arteries have narrowed or who has already suffered a "ministroke" or a TIA (transient ischemic attack).

So put this in your nonforgettable memory compartment. If you can't remember where that is, ask your wife. She'll know for sure. Symptoms that require immediate attention include:

- a sudden very severe headache (not your usual migraine but the kind of headache that is described as the worst you could have)
- sudden difficulty speaking or understanding speech (except, I suppose, when listening to sports announcers)
- sudden loss of vision
- sudden weakness or paralysis in a limb or facial muscles
- sudden dizziness and confusion

All these symptoms should be treated as an emergency. Happily, many times, the cause of these symptoms will not be a stroke, but never take that chance.

CHAPTER 6

Plan A: You Are What You Eat and Drink

If I had known that I was going to live this long,
I would have taken better care of myself.

—MICKEY MANTLE

Not only do persons with better health habits survive longer, disability is
postponed and compressed into fewer years at the end of life.

—ANTHONY J. VITA, et al., *New England Journal of Medicine*

Trying in my usual gentle manner to make a point one day, I asked one of the nonmedical reviewers of this text if he had been struck by the connection among the chronic health problems discussed in the preceding chapter. The immediate reply was, "Sure, man. They're all things that only happen to you when you're really old, man. Like over fifty." Not for the first time did it occur to me that things might work much better if teenage sons and their fathers inhabited separate planets.

"No," I persisted. "What I meant is that all those diseases are nearly entirely preventable if you do all the right things starting early in life."

"There you go again, Dad," came the reply. "As usual, you're trying to turn everything into a lecture. I'm outta here, man."

Lecture? Is that what this reads like, I wondered for a few seconds before dismissing his clearly inaccurate assessment and banning him from using the car for a month. But his words do lead me to make this disclaimer: none of this should read like a lecture for the simple reason that lectures about lifestyle never alter behaviour. All I want, all

I really, really want, is to point out how the choices you have already made might affect you and what you can do to minimize certain health risks. Then you can decide what to do with that information.

So let me start by telling you that a study in the *Journal of the American Medical Association* concluded that death in old age is never the result of only one cause. Rather, we tend to die as a result of several underlying factors that are a product of "lifelong habits," which can largely be changed.

The good news is that to a certain extent, we are getting the message. A U.S. study has concluded that disabilities in seniors dropped by 14.5 per cent between 1982 and 1994. And men seem to be getting the message more clearly than women. For example, although in most western countries and most cultures women have been outliving men by an average of 7 to 8 years, according to Canadian government statistics, the difference in life expectancy between men and women in Canada had actually shrunk to 5.9 years by 1995, mostly because men's improved lifestyles have resulted in a more rapid decrease in deaths from heart attacks and strokes among men than among women.

In case any of you guys are tempted to rest on your laurels, however, don't, because we could all still be doing much better.

So this chapter is devoted to trying to get you to change to a more healthy lifestyle, because, according to a study in the *New England Journal of Medicine*, "Persons with better health habits survive longer [and] disability is postponed and compressed into fewer years at the end of life."

An important caveat, however. As you will quickly notice, I have been very selective in the bits that I discuss. Thus, I will not discuss the need to avoid too much sun exposure (self-evident) or the hazards of recreational drugs. Nor will I spend much effort discussing the need to stop smoking, because I give you some credit: if you are still using drugs or smoking by middle age, you no doubt know exactly what you're doing, to yourself and to those around you, and I doubt that anything I say is going to get through to you. Now that doesn't sound much like a lecture, does it?

You will also notice that I have divided healthy lifestyle habits into two chapters. This chapter discusses things you should and should not ingest, while the second deals with all the other issues of healthy living. Why the split? Because the lifestyle habits discussed in this chapter are the ones I consider the easiest habits to alter, since they don't involve any active work, something nearly all of us, me included, try to avoid as much as possible. The lifestyle habits described in Chapter 7, however, require much more effort. But those habits are probably also the ones that will have the greatest effect on your health.

DIET

Most of us, especially you, eat too much, and this is not good for you. For example, when researchers reduced the food intake of lab rats by 30 to 40 per cent, the rats extended their life-spans by one-third. (This finding also explains why there are so many old, thin lawyers around.) What is true for rats is equally true for humans. According to no less an authority than the *New England Journal of Medicine*, "calorie restriction slows age-related deficits in behavior, learning, immune response, gene expression, and DNA repair," a lot of deficits you would really like to avoid because they probably shorten your life expectancy, not to mention how much they affect the quality of your life.

We also don't eat regularly enough. What Mom told you is really true. Breakfast is important. A British study concluded that people who eat breakfast foods, especially cereals, tend to eat fewer fatty foods the rest of the day. The researchers also claim that breakfast eaters tend to get a healthy serving of fibre and vitamins from their breakfast foods, although the researchers clearly did not mean those who eat the typical British breakfast of three fried eggs, complemented with that acme of British cuisine, four slices of fried bread.

Most important, however, we also eat too much of the wrong foods and don't eat enough of the right ones. Thus, an international panel of experts recently claimed that 30 to 40 per cent of all cancers could be avoided if people ate a healthier diet (and got enough exercise).

What kind of foods am I talking about? Simple. We ingest too much protein, sugar, and refined carbohydrates, but most of all we ingest far too much saturated fat. If you make only one change to your diet after reading this section, cut down on your intake of saturated fat.

But while saturated fat is bad, bad, bad, polyunsaturated fats and especially, perhaps, mono-unsaturated fats are not as bad and may even be good for you. In one study that particularly appeals to this lover of Greek food, a Mediterranean diet, which is high in mono-unsaturated fat, especially olive oil, lowered the risk of a second heart attack in men who had already had one heart attack by over 75 per cent over two years.

You should also probably pay some attention to the trans-fatty acids in partially hydrogenated vegetable oils, the types of fats in all those high-fat, high-calorie foods such as potato chips and packaged cookies, as well as in hard margarines. Studies have suggested that trans-fatty acids are even worse for you than saturated fats.

And if you do still have to eat some saturated fats, such as dairy products, for their calcium content, try to substitute low-fat or nonfat products for those containing whole fats. As to how you find a low-fat T-bone steak, I'm afraid I don't have any good suggestions for you.

I realize that this is all much easier said than done, and I know that no matter what the evidence shows and no matter how much I exhort you, many of us, including me, will find it very difficult to abandon our prime rib and baked potato with sour cream for breast of tofu swathed in olive oil and low-fat yogurt. So here's something to chew on, guys. Get some help, because the research shows that men whose wives support their effort to stick to dietary changes are much more likely to succeed. After all, every convict needs a good warden to keep him on the path to righteousness.

For the more determined of you, keep in mind that you don't have to go whole hog. One popular way to eat fewer saturated fats, at least among today's teenagers, is to become a vegetarian, and a vegetarian diet is indeed generally very healthy. A study from New Zealand found that vegetarians have an up to 40 per cent lower risk of dying from heart disease and cancer than meat eaters.

Sounds great, but as usual, there are some cautions. First, many people who set out to become vegetarians don't stick with it for very long. Second, although vegetarians don't die as much from heart disease and cancer, they are much more likely than meat eaters to die of boredom and violent death, the latter from the huge risk vegetarians run of being shot by a meat-eating friend who has prepared a dinner of Chateaubriand for them.

Third, a vegetarian diet may be bad for your brain. According to one theory, the move away from a vegetarian diet is what allowed our ancestors' brains to grow. In other words, it wasn't an apple that the snake gave Eve, it was a burger. This theory postulates that once they were freed of the need to use so much energy to digest the vast amounts of rabbit food necessary to stem their hunger, early man and woman could use more energy to think. Thus, meat equalled wisdom, while veggies equalled lack of same. As evidence that these equations still hold, I point to an American survey that found that self-proclaimed vegetarians ate more fish and poultry over a two-week test period than did self-proclaimed carnivores. Dumb and dumber.

As to the foods you should eat more of, I want to stress fibre, because fibre lowers the risk of many common illnesses linked to our western way of life, such as, among other things:

- appendicitis
- diverticulosis (intestinal outpouchings that are subject to inflammation and infection)
- heart disease
- colon polyps and colon cancer
- hemorrhoids
- irritable bowel syndrome
- Type II diabetes
- high blood pressure
- gallstones

A word to the wise, however. Introduce fibre to your diet in small increments. Your bowel needs to get used to an increased amount of fibre. If you introduce it too quickly, your bowel will signal its displeasure the only way a bowel can. Man the lifeboats, and try to work alone that day.

You should also increase the amount of fish you eat, especially oily fish, such as salmon and even mackerel. It has been shown that Japanese who never eat fish have a 32 per cent higher mortality rate from all causes than those who eat fish daily, and those numbers would be even more in favour of the fish eaters, I think, if the Japanese didn't also have a nasty habit of eating fish and fish products (like fugu) that can kill you instantly. (My son has a theory that whatever we non-Japanese consider disgusting, the Japanese consider a delicacy, and I have not yet been able to prove him wrong.) The only drawback to eating more fish is a slightly higher risk of clotting abnormalities (fish oils prevent clotting), perhaps a slightly deleterious effect on LDL levels, and possibly a tendency to develop gills.

You should also eat loads of fruits and veggies. They contain gobs of antioxidant vitamins such as vitamins C and E, and beta-carotene. Antioxidants mop up harmful chemicals called free radicals, those Abby Hoffman dirty little buggers that are produced by oxygenation reactions in the body and that lead to degenerative diseases and aging. Eating a wide range and abundance of fruits and vegetables (and beans and grains) will also provide you with lots of other important compounds linked to lower rates of all sorts of diseases. These compounds include complex carbohydrates, flavonoids, sulforaphane, and phenols, among many others.

Many more foods and beverages have been promoted by health-food nuts for their health effects, such as brown rice, garlic, brewer's yeast, kelp, and a host of others. If you can enjoy a kelp and nettle stew, all power to you (but don't invite me for dinner; I have other plans that night, namely, surviving). I do, however, want to make a note of two foods and one beverage that I am partial to. Drink more tea (which contains lots of antioxidants), and eat more nuts (which contain a good kind of fat) and raisins (which may help lower cholesterol levels).

One food I do not push much, however, is tofu. Although every food expert in the world wants you to eat more soy (which acts like estrogen on the tissues), a "soybering" study on Hawaiian men found that those who ate the most soy had the highest rate and most severe cases of Alzheimer's disease—which brings me to this editorial comment. Hard as this is to accept in our one-stop world, there is no magic food. Not tofu, not kelp, not even yogurt, which has long been touted as the main reason all those Azerbaijani centenarians live to their ripe old age. But according to a recent story by a reporter who went to the valley where all those old people live, many of them hate yogurt. Never eat the stuff. So we've had it backwards all along. Maybe avoiding yogurt is what can help you live longer.

Finally, even if you don't want to change your diet at all, there may still be hope for you, because a California-based company claims it's soon going to market veggies in pill form. I can hardly wait.

SUPPLEMENTS, MINERALS, HERBS

Let me first put my bias squarely on the table. Although I strongly believe in God, country, Manchester United, the Habs, roast chicken, peaches, and pike and carp for gefilte fish (although not necessarily in that order), I don't believe in most supplements, because I just can't see that in a world that gives us cashews and cantaloupe and cauliflower and Camembert that God or Darwin ever intended for us to swallow a bunch of capsules every day instead of eating enough of the real stuff the capsules are intended to mimic. It's only our misplaced arrogance piled on top of our sloth that has allowed an industry of supplement pushers to sprout and bloom and convince us of the lifesaving properties of their overpriced potions. It's not that supplements can't do you some good. Many do, and some do a lot of good. But many of the claims made on behalf of supplements are at best premature and at worst self-serving exaggerations meant to dull the public's much more urgent need to change its lifestyle for the better. Taking vitamins E and C and beta-carotene and ginseng and lecithin and garlic capsules every day is never going to do you as much good as getting enough exercise and following a healthy, well-balanced diet.

Now that I have vented my spleen, I will be more rational and say that so long as you are following a healthy lifestyle, there are a couple of supplements that I think might be beneficial for you, although the people who take the most supplements are usually the people who need them least.

Vitamins
So let's get the rah-rah stuff out of the way first. Most studies have shown that people who either take vitamin supplements or have higher blood levels of certain vitamins, especially the antioxidant vitamins C and E and the carotene family (precursors of vitamin A), are in better health than those who don't. To list all the studies that show a positive effect from higher levels of antioxidants in the blood is impossible, so let me just highlight a few of the important ones for us guys, some of which have been covered previously.

In a Finnish study, smoking men—that is, men who smoke, not men on fire—who took small doses of vitamin E reduced their risk of getting prostate cancer by 30 per cent and reduced their risk of dying from prostate cancer by over 40 per cent. Vitamin E has also been linked to a lower risk of colon cancer and coronary heart disease and a slower progression of Alzheimer's disease, and in elderly people, vitamin E boosts immunity.

Lycopene, a member of the carotene family, seems to help prevent prostate and colorectal cancer and perhaps coronary heart disease.

Studies suggest that folate and vitamin B_6 lower the risk of heart attack and that vitamin C exerts a protective effect on the arteries of diabetics. Middling to high doses of vitamin C and beta-carotene, as well as higher doses of vitamin D, have been linked to a lower risk of osteoarthritis and less pain should the osteoarthritis occur. Vitamin C might inhibit the growth of the bacteria linked to peptic ulcers. A higher intake of antioxidant vitamins has also been linked to lower risks of cataracts and age-related macular degeneration, the most common cause of blindness in the elderly, and to a lower risk of recurrence of polyps in the colon, precursors to cancer (see Chapter 8).

There is lots more, but most of you are already no doubt screaming, "Enough already. Isn't it clear? We should all be taking extra daily hits of multi-vitamins." You may be right, especially since it's very hard to get enough of two of the most important vitamins, vitamin E and folic acid, from the diet. But as a cautious doctor who has seen far too much medical gold turn into lead, I have to urge caution because there are still some solid objections to counselling the widespread use of supplements.

First, pushing supplements deflects attention from the need to make all the other proven-to-be-beneficial though harder-to-stick-to lifestyle adjustments. Second, it is probably not a good idea to single out one or two vitamins that people should take because it's more likely that the greatest benefit to health lies in the proper balance of all nutrients, and overdosing on one or two may skew that balance. We simply have no idea how different doses of these vitamins interact or what doses are required to get a desired health effect. Finally, there's the very important fact that even vitamins are not without known risk. Here are just a few examples:

- A huge study on the effect of supplements on cancer was halted early when it was discovered that the men taking beta-carotene were dying more rapidly than were the non–vitamin takers.
- In a Finnish study cited earlier, men on beta-carotene had a higher risk of prostate cancer than men on placebo.
- In most studies involving vitamin E, the risk of cerebral hemorrhage went up with increasing doses of the vitamin.
- High doses of vitamin C have been linked to a higher risk of kidney stones.

The point of all these objections is that although vitamins may be natural, so is arsenic. Natural can still be unhealthy, especially in large doses, and we just don't know enough yet to advise everyone to take lots more supplements.

One other important note: no matter what bill of goods your local health food store might try to sell you, there is no proof that for most purposes, the much more expensive "natural-source" vitamins are any better than the synthetic vitamins, at least not better for you. They are certainly better for the bottom line of the people trying to sell you these overpriced panaceas.

Calcium

A middle-aged man needs about 1000 mg of calcium per day, and if you simply cannot get enough from your diet—if, for example, you don't particularly like salmon bones and whey—then by all means take calcium supplements. My experience has been that all forms of calcium supplements take a bit of getting used to, but on the whole calcium citrate is less likely to cause stomach upset than the other forms.

DHEA (Dehydroepiandrosterone)

Although DHEA is not legally available in Canada, it has still become the supplement du jour in North America. I sincerely hope that unlike melatonin and tryptophan and several others, DHEA is not largely forgotten when the new chemical boy comes to town. For now, however, DHEA, a hormone produced in the adrenal glands and a precursor to both androgens and estrogen, is king. And why not? Get a load of what its proponents claim that DHEA can do. It may:

- improve immune function
- inhibit clotting
- lower the risk of coronary heart disease
- lower the risk of some cancers
- protect against Type II diabetes
- help prevent lupus
- postpone signs of aging
- prevent a loss of libido
- help impotence
- help elevate mood
- lead to a greater ability to cope with stressful events
- lead to less depression
- increase muscle strength
- increase physical mobility
- make bodies leaner
- promote deeper and more restorative sleep

And I'll bet some people claim that it helps you play the piano too.

Even a golden boy has some potential flaws, however, so be aware that some experts believe that DHEA might provoke a latent prostate cancer to grow more quickly. Sit tight on that for a while.

Echinacea

An old joke:

Doctor: "Take this pill, Jack, and your cold will be gone in seven days."

Jack: "And if I do nothing, doc?"

Doc: "Then you'll be better in a week."

Echinacea, a herb, is widely promoted for boosting immunity, especially to prevent or treat the symptoms of a cold, so what I am about to say is unlikely to dissuade true believers from using echinacea the next time they come down with the sniffles. But a double-blind Canadian study involving several hundred students found that the students on echinacea felt better in about a week. Case closed.

Garlic

Among the claims made for garlic, all of which are disputed by other studies, the main ones concern its ability to help the heart and the arteries. Thus, it is claimed that garlic can make arteries more flexible, that it can prevent clotting, and that it lowers blood pressure and cholesterol levels. In addition, a U.S. study found that garlic prevented the growth of tumours in mice, although there was one major complication in this regime. You see, the garlic-eating mice quickly lost all their friends.

Ginkgo Biloba

A very much-hyped study found that extracts of ginkgo biloba improved cognitive performance in some Alzheimer's patients. So I am sure that many of you will be spurred to run out and buy some ginkgo, if you can remember what to buy, that is, or why you went to the store in the first place.

Selenium

This supplement is probably the least appreciated and may turn out to be the most valuable one in the end. A study in the *Journal of the American Medical Association* found that after subjects used 200 mg of selenium daily for four and a half years, the incidence of cancer for all subjects was reduced by 50 per cent, especially for prostate cancer, colon cancer, and lung cancer.

Zinc
Several studies have found that zinc can boost immunity and may be especially helpful in preventing colds and flus. Conversely, too much zinc can impair immunity and lower HDL levels.

Finally, the million-dollar question: what do I, the conservative, skeptical author, do? I take daily doses of vitamin E, folic acid, and calcium, of course. Hey! You gotta hedge your bets.

ASA (Acetylsalicylic Acid)

This is one pill I like, especially for preventing heart attacks. Although many men who are not at high risk of heart attack take ASA every day, this practice has proven to be most effective in high-risk men, such as those who have already had a heart attack or those with established coronary heart disease. As for lower-risk men, there is one study on male doctors in which ASA was shown to prevent heart attacks in normal-risk men too, but this is still a hot issue in medical circles.

The reason I like ASA is that it seems to have other health benefits as well. Regular ASA use has been linked to a lower risk of colon cancer, and taking nonsteroidal anti-inflammatories regularly has been linked to a lower risk of Alzheimer's disease. Since ASA is the champion nonsteroidal anti-inflammatory, we're left with the inescapable conclusion that everyone should be taking an ASA every day, right? Well, as my chummy professors used to yell at me as I headed out the door well before the lecture was over, "Not so quick, you there. Not so quick." The following factors may mitigate against taking an ASA every day:

- Although regular use of other nonsteroidal anti-inflammatories (such as ibuprofen) has been linked to a lower risk of Alzheimer's disease, ASA has not as yet.
- We still don't know if ASA does much good for men who have a healthy lifestyle most of the time.
- ASA can produce bothersome side effects, most notably gastrointestinal disturbances such as an upset stomach and nausea.

- ASA is linked to a higher risk of stomach ulcers, which not only can cause pain but can also bleed and even hemorrhage and rupture. This risk can be lowered, happily, but not eliminated, by using enteric-coated ASA or other stomach-protecting medications.
- Anyone at risk of a bleeding problem puts himself at even higher risk if he also starts to take ASA regularly, since ASA inhibits clotting. Thus, regular use of ASA increases the risk of dying from a cerebral hemorrhage. Although the overall risk of cerebral hemorrhage is much lower than the overall risk of a heart attack, it is still of concern for men at high risk of this deadly complication, such as men with high blood pressure.

If you decide to take ASA daily, one other problem you run into is that doctors still don't know which dose of ASA is best. The less you take the better, of course, but only if you take enough of it to do you some good. And according to a recent study, low doses of ASA may just not work as well as hoped. In this study, men on low doses of ASA required twice monthly boosters with a hit of super-strength ASA in order for the ASA to maintain its anticlotting properties.

Perhaps the best news, then, is that a super-ASA is on its way. This new type of ASA, at regular doses, is not only much more effective at doing all the good stuff ASA does but is also much less likely to irritate the stomach or damage the kidneys.

Finally, a potentially very important health benefit of ASA: ASA can be lifesaving if you think you are having a heart attack or if you are at high risk for a heart attack and are suddenly catapulted into an extremely stressful situation, such as waking up to an earthquake or coming home to find your wife gone, your house stripped bare, and a note on the floor with your name on it. Downing a prophylactic ASA immediately in those situations can save your life by preventing a blood clot from forming in the first place or by preventing a small clot from getting larger. It won't bring back the couch or lamps, but it will better your chances to live and fight in court another day.

ALCOHOL

I can think of no better way to start a discussion of alcohol than with a glass, or preferably two, of a nice manly yet mellow Merlot. Or, if you're a wuss, perhaps a Chardonnay. Actually, given my very low tolerance for alcohol, after two glasses, I usually can't even tell if it was a red or a white I had started out drinking. Or if it was even wine.

Although it's not at all a unanimous view, many experts believe that a "moderate" intake of alcohol is good for most of you and an "excess" is very bad. But how good is "good"? To borrow from the evangelists: Good Is Great. And it seems to be equally great everywhere we look. Thus, according to a huge long-term study by researchers at the American Cancer Society, overall death rates—deaths from all causes—were lowest among those who drank one alcoholic drink a day.

A study from the Department of Public Health in Perth, Australia, found that the risk of mortality from all causes is about 15 per cent lower for people who drink some alcohol than for nondrinkers. And I think this study is well worth paying attention to, since Australians know more than most about alcohol. You could be stuck in the tiniest village in the remotest outcrop of an island on the coldest continent, but if you stumble into the moonshiner's kitchen, odds are that the first words you will hear will be the only other patron saying, "G'day, mate. Buyin' the next round?"

A study from England found that the "healthiest" group comprised nonsmokers drinking 20 to 29 units of alcohol (one unit = one glass of wine, one small bottle or can of beer, or a one-ounce shot of hard liquor) each week, while a Danish study concluded that drinking both red and white wine was associated with lower death rates overall in men between thirty and seventy.

And finally, there's the French. Now the French clearly see the world somewhat differently from you and me. I mean, French folk treat Jerry Lewis as an icon, for Pete's sake.

So it's certainly possible that the French might gather and interpret their statistics a bit differently than we do. Nonetheless, most experts still agree that despite doing few of the things we think are essential to prevent heart disease, the population in parts of France has lower levels of heart disease-related mortality than we do in North America— the famous French paradox. When I say that the French don't try to protect their hearts, here is what I mean. In North America, the experts tell us that if we want to protect our hearts, we have to avoid smoking, avoid cholesterol and saturated fats, and do some aerobic exercise. And how do the French treat that advice? With a Gallic shrug, of course. As a frequent tourist to France, I can tell you that just by walking into a Paris bistro, restaurant, or pub, you have passively inhaled one pack of Gauloises before you even hit your seat (next to a woman with a poodle named Chou-Chou on her lap, no doubt); that if you ask a Frenchman where you can find a low-cholesterol or low-fat meal, he will invariably smirk and point to England; and that the French do absolutely no aerobic exercise—after all, has anyone ever seen any Frenchman run?

So what protects the French from an epidemic of heart disease? Most experts agree that it must at least in part be their alcohol intake, and to that end the French are great suppliers of statistics backing up this view. An excellent example is a recent report in the journal *Epidemiology* that followed 34,000 Frenchmen for fifteen years and found that moderate wine drinkers had a 20 per cent lower risk of death from cancer than all other groups and a 20 to 30 per cent reduced risk of heart attack and brain hemorrhage, or stroke.

So experts everywhere agree: moderate alcohol intake can help you live longer. Besides its beneficial effect on life expectancy, though, moderate alcohol intake may exert other positive health benefits as well.

- A study from Boston on male physicians found that moderate alcohol intake (how come doctors are always so willing to take part in studies on alcohol?) lowered the risk of a second heart attack in those men who had already had one heart attack or stroke.
- Wine may protect your stomach against infection. In the lab, at any rate, wine did a better job of killing off bacteria such as *E. coli*, *Shigella*, or *Salmonella*, common causes of food poisoning and that scourge known as turista, than did the commonly prescribed remedy, Pepto-Bismol. So the next time I go to Mexico, to hell with all the preventive antibiotics. Some Merlot by the minute, and hey, even if I get turista, I won't mind.
- Moderate alcohol consumption has been associated with a decreased risk of *H. pylori* infection, the bacteria that causes gastritis and peptic ulcers.
- Wine drinking has also been linked to lower rates of age-related macular degeneration, the leading cause of blindness in the elderly, as well as a lower risk of kidney stones.
- According to a study in the *Journal of Wine Research* (and I'm sure these guys have absolutely no bias), red wine can even help you

recover from radiation poisoning. So if you happen to get caught in a nuclear war, just remember to get hold of a few bottles of plonk, and I'm sure all will end well.

- Finally, as Ogden Nash pointed out, "Candy, /Is dandy,/But Liquor, /Is quicker." A study from Finland concluded that two glasses of wine has an aphrodisiac effect on women, probably because alcohol raises testosterone levels in women. There was no equivalent effect on men, however.

All in all, then, moderate alcohol intake seems to be correlated not only with a longer life but also with a better quality of life. But how, you may well wonder, does alcohol exert its positive effect? We don't know, but as usual, there are lots of theories:

- Moderate amounts of alcohol raise the levels of HDL.
- Alcohol may also lower LDL levels a bit in some men (although it may have a slightly deleterious effect on triglyceride levels).
- Alcohol may slow clotting of the blood.
- Some substances in alcohol have antioxidant effects.
- It has also been postulated that the substance in red wine known as resveratrol has an estrogenlike protective effect on tissues such as the heart and the brain.
- My theory is that alcohol exerts at least some of its positive effects because it lowers anxiety levels. After all, a couple of glasses of wine and even your teenagers seem manageable.

The most likely explanation, however, is some sort of combination of all of the above.

But that brings us to this important question: how does "moderate" alcohol intake differ from "excess"? I have always believed, and told my patients, that "excess alcohol intake" is simply "anything more than I drink." A more objective answer is that moderate alcohol intake is one to three glasses of wine—or the equivalent amount of alcohol in other spirits—per day on most days. Not everyone agrees with this guideline, however.

On the one hand, a long-term study of physicians found that those male doctors who had two to four drinks a *week* had the lowest overall rate of death from all causes and that those who drank over one glass of alcohol a day had no increased life expectancy over teetotallers.

On the other hand, the Danish study I referred to earlier found that three to five glasses of wine a day was correlated with the best health.

So which is it? Well, even if the Danes are right, I think that three to five glasses of wine a day is simply too much to aim for, and certainly too much to recommend to the public, because we live in a society where most people believe that "if a little of something I like is good, a whole lot must be even better." So if we gave the green light to men to consume up to five glasses of wine or five beers a day guilt-free, many men would take that as tacit permission to drink even more (many already do), and they would consequently leave themselves open to all the problems excess alcohol intake leads to. I prefer to err on the side of caution and say that one to three glasses of wine a day is the maximum to consume regularly.

So much for alcohol's potential benefits. What about—the teetotallers are no doubt bursting to shout—alcohol's negative health effects, especially those on the brain? After all, alcohol is a powerful toxin and even a small amount of alcohol is bound to kill some brain cells.

Not in Scandinavia, however. According to a study from Denmark in which the brains of alcoholics were analyzed (at autopsy, I hope; I mean even in laid-back Denmark I'm sure they couldn't get away with doing it the other way) and compared with the brains of nondrinkers, there was no detectable difference between the two groups in number of neurons in the neocortex, the part of the brain associated with higher brain functions such as remembering where to find the Little Mermaid. There is one teeny caveat to all this, however, because when compared with teetotallers' brains, drinkers' brains were "shrunken" in other areas, such as those involved in sexual response, anger, fight-or-flight, and fear, a finding that could go a long way in explaining why men who drink a lot are always ready to challenge all comers that theirs is bigger than yours. It's not, but hey, that's usually not the time or the place to argue.

Alcohol doesn't seem to hurt Australian brains, either. A study of Australian veterans found that long-term moderate use of alcohol did not impair cognitive functions, although I am amazed that they were able to find Aussie soldiers who drank only moderately.

As to other tissues, such as bones, muscles, and internal organs, in moderate amounts, alcohol seems to have few negative effects.

As for which type of alcohol is best, most studies claim to find only slight differences between equivalent amounts of wine and beer and to a lesser extent, hard liquor. As a committed wine drinker and a equally committed beer hater, however, I have to say that a good Merlot or Cabernet Sauvignon will clearly beat a bottled Bud every time. Thus, I prefer studies such as the one from Denmark I cited earlier, in which beer drinkers were not nearly as likely to benefit from their alcohol intake as were the winers like me, or a study from the University of North Carolina that found that drink for drink, beer guzzlers and hard-liquor drinkers were three times as likely to have a larger waist-to-hip ratio than wine drinkers. Since a high waist-to-hip ratio is correlated with higher rates of cardiac disease (see the section on weight in Chapter 7), winers' lower waist-to-hip ratio may help explain why they are better off than those big-butted, fat-waisted, couthless, smelly beer guzzlers.

Before you get carried away with the benefits of alcohol, however, remember this important caution: Ten to 20 per cent of the population cannot handle alcohol at all, and if you're one of those people, stay away from this (for you) very dangerous substance. Do not be seduced by the glowing reports of alcohol's benefits. They don't apply to you because alcoholics are much more likely to suffer the negative consequences of alcohol well before the positive ones kick in. And alcoholism is a lifelong disease that requires lifelong therapy, which consists of the avoidance of alcohol. Even if you don't consider yourself an alcoholic, you must still remember that a lot of alcohol is definitely not better than a little. Excess alcohol intake is related to a higher level of:

- heart attacks
- several cancers
- cirrhosis
- impotence
- neurological disorders
- depression
- sleep disorders

In addition, excess alcohol intake is associated with much higher rates of death from suicide and accidents, not to mention that you often can't walk straight and you generally smell like hell, too.

Remember too that alcohol interacts with many medications, and it may be especially dangerous when you are also taking analgesics such as ASA, acetaminophen, and other over-the-counter painkillers. This potentially lethal combo has been linked to a higher risk of liver damage, bleeding from the stomach, and sudden death.

Also—and this is very important—don't binge. Regular, daily intake may be healthy for you, but bingeing is most assuredly not. Middle-aged Finnish men who binge on beer, which for this study's purposes was taken as a six-pack or more at one sitting, were found to have a much greater risk of having a fatal heart attack and of dying violently than men who drink less than three bottles per session.

If you don't already drink, there is absolutely no evidence that you should suddenly start drinking as soon as you finish this chapter (or sooner). Not only do teetotallers do pretty well in many studies, but there is also no proof that suddenly starting to drink alcohol in your middle years after a lifetime of abstention is going to help you live longer and better, although it will probably permit you to have more fun.

Finally, this editorial comment: not only does excess alcohol intake often ruin the life of the drinker, but it often ruins the lives of his or her family members as well, and not just in the obvious ways. If you are drinking too much—and there are all sorts of self-administered tests and quizzes available on the Internet and from drug-and-alcohol agencies and health professionals to help you determine if you have a problem with alcohol—then for your own sake as well as that of your family, friends, co-workers, and potential victims, seek some professional help. But seek it from a professional who knows what he or she is doing. Your old family doctor may not, I'm afraid, be the best person to help you unless she is also prepared to be very honest and harsh and also willing and able to take the considerable amount of time needed to deal with you and your games.

Having said all that, one last word: *l'chaim!*

CAFFEINE

Some sour souls have become captive to a hatred of caffeine, and especially coffee, that defies all rational explanation. Now that the war on tobacco is nearly won, I am sure these zealots will turn their guns on caffeine so that we will soon, I fear, be witness to all sorts of restrictive anticoffee laws, such as not being allowed to drink coffee in public buildings or restaurants except in special decaf sections, or even in planes ("this airplane is equipped with the latest coffee detectors in the washrooms, and anyone found drinking coffee will be thrown out in midflight"), all of which will no doubt be preceded by studies showing the terrible consequences of secondhand coffee intake. "Our study found that 80 per cent of mellow people sitting next to someone drinking a double cappuccino report becoming jumpy."

It is these coffee haters, I'm sure, who are behind all those studies that have claimed that coffee is responsible for deleterious health consequences such as

- elevated cholesterol levels
- an increased risk of heart attack
- an increased risk of cancer of the pancreas
- osteoporosis
- a rise in blood pressure
- all sorts of mental, psychological, and physiological impairments, such as a decreased ability to think and concentrate as well as poorer performance on many tasks

To the chagrin of the coffee haters, however, nearly all those "bad-coffee" findings have been flushed away in subsequent follow-up studies. Moderate amounts of coffee are *not associated* with increased risks of osteoporosis, heart attack (although it can raise blood pressure a bit), or cancer, nor does it impair performance of any sort.

As far as science can tell (and I'm sure this galls the coffee haters), if you are a healthy person, coffee in moderate amounts is not bad for you, and even if you're not healthy, it's unlikely that moderate amounts of coffee will do you much harm. What may be even more disheartening to anticoffee nuts, however, is that if you are not already jiving with java, perhaps you should be. Here are some of the benefits of coffee:

- An excellent way for long-distance travellers to ease their jet lag is to force themselves to wake up at the appropriate hour in their new time zone and drink a couple of strong cuppas.
- Caffeine perks you up—it stimulates the central nervous system, producing a heightened sense of alertness, faster thinking, and an increased ability to pay attention (in between extra visits to the washroom, of course) while also minimizing fatigue.

- Caffeine dilates arteries to the heart—although I would still recommend that you take an ASA instead of making a quick visit to a Starbuck's at the first sign of a heart attack.
- Caffeine constricts arteries to the head, meaning that caffeine is useful as a headache remedy.
- Caffeine may even help lower the risk of bowel cancer, perhaps because caffeine speeds transit time through the bowel. The bowel, like a commuter on his twice-daily cross-town commute, much prefers a rapid transit time.
- Another benefit for a steak lover like me is that according to Swiss researchers, coffee can neutralize cancer-causing chemicals in well-done meat.
- And British researchers have found that drinking coffee can counter the effects of having a cold.
- Perhaps caffeine's most important health benefit, though, is that as several studies have shown, caffeine drinkers are less prone to depression and suicide. Why? In part, I suppose, because coffee drinkers are too hyper to kill themselves but probably also because coffee has a positive effect on brain chemicals such as serotonin.

Reluctantly, I must admit that coffee does have a bad side:

- Coffee before exercise can boost both systolic and diastolic blood pressure readings for up to forty minutes, mostly in men who are already hypertensive, but also to an extent in healthy men. So you probably don't want to combine a jug of java with a jog.
- Also, a Danish study found that drinking five or more cups of coffee a day may increase levels of homocysteine in the blood. The problem with this study, however, is that the Danes tend to drink unfiltered coffee with their herring and pastries, so these results may apply only to that kind of coffee or even to that kind of combination.
- There's also the problem of caffeine withdrawal, which is usually associated with headache and lethargy. That is why those people who drown themselves in coffee during the week but who swear off coffee on weekends to "relax" often spend the weekend making the rest of us feel more tense.
- Perhaps coffee's best-known deleterious effect, though, is its tendency to interfere with sleep, as do the many over-the-counter

painkillers that contain caffeine. That late-night cup of French roast can also increase symptoms of gastroesophageal reflux disease.

Happily, though, even these seemingly intrusive side effects can have an unintended positive consequence; at least one study has shown that seniors who drink coffee at night have more sex than seniors who don't drink coffee. Well, if you're going to be up late at night, how much Leno or Letterman can you watch anyway?

Finally, if you haven't yet learned to love coffee by the time you're fifty, I don't suppose that you ought to start drinking it now, even if it is bloody time you stopped being so damn mellow. Sorry about that. A little caffeine jumpiness there, I'm afraid.

CHAPTER 7

Plan B: The Harder Work Involved in Becoming Healthy

The wise for cure on exercise depend.

—JOHN DRYDEN

Early to rise and early to bed
makes a male healthy and wealthy and dead.

—JAMES THURBER, "The Shrike and the Chipmunks," *Fables for Our Time*

OK, guys. I hope you've rested and recovered from reading that last chapter and that you're ready to plough on because I have some bad news for you. Chapter 6 was what I consider to be the easy stuff on how to stay healthy. After all, anyone can change his or her diet a bit, especially if it doesn't involve eating tofu, and most of you will also have very little trouble, I'm sure, drinking a few more cappuccinos and an extra glass or two of wine every day. But the sad fact is that even if you make all the changes I recommend in Chapter 6, that will still not be enough to much improve your chances of living longer and better.

I know most of you don't want to hear this but it takes more than just changing what and how you chew or swallow to maximize your chances of being healthy when you hit your older years. It actually takes some effort. You can't get very healthy, I'm afraid, by just sitting on the couch or at the dining room table. And that's what this chapter is dedicated to—some of the harder work involved in improving your lifestyle. You must start to pay more attention to your weight, to your sleeping habits, and to your stress level, and most important, you must become more active.

"But why now?" you may well whine to your mate when she reads you this bit. "Why is Hister bugging me to become more active at this time in my life? Why not wait till I'm just a bit older, like seventy-eight, perhaps, before I start trying to stop the clock?" The answer to that is simple: because midlife is when it's best to make healthy changes to your lifestyle. The Honolulu Heart Program, for example, has concluded that although it's never too late to change, you get the biggest bang for your buck if you make the appropriate lifestyle adjustments in midlife.

WEIGHT

A quick look around you will reveal that overall we who live in the developed nations are avoiring too much dupois, and we're padding that dupois with unseemly alacrity. Surveys reveal that more than two-thirds of American adults weigh more than is recommended for their height and age, and that about half are obese, or at least 20 per cent over their ideal weight. Although as usual, the Americans are out in front of the rest of us, especially their profiles, the sad fact is that every developed nation is heading for a mountain of trouble from the legions of bowling-ball-shaped baby boomers plodding and shuffling into their dotage.

Why is excess weight bad for you? Because it can kill you. A study that looked at Harvard alumni for over thirty years, for example, found a "straight line" relationship between weight and mortality; men who weighed 20 per cent less than the average for their height had the lowest mortality rate, whereas men who were obese had the highest mortality rate.

And being overweight in midlife is probably worse than being overweight at any other time. There is some proof, for example, that being somewhat overweight when you're older is not only not bad for you, it may even signal good health, probably because one of the first things that happens to most elderly people when they become sick is losing some weight. This is certainly not the case with younger adults, however. Thus, the risk of coronary heart disease in middle age is related to excess weight, and this risk seems to remain higher even if the excess weight is eventually taken off, which is why a study from the University of Buffalo found that middle-aged men who were overweight when the study began had a higher overall death rate at all ages, especially from heart disease, than men who were not overweight.

How does excess weight kill? Mostly through its deleterious effect on the heart and cardiovascular system. Several studies, including the fifty-year-long Framingham study, have revealed that obese people end up with higher blood pressure, larger hearts, and thicker walls in the pumping chambers of the heart, all of which are linked to an increased risk of premature disease and death.

Even a small increase in weight can raise your risk of having a heart attack, even if you have no other risk factors for coronary heart disease. The Female Nurses' Health Study, for example, found that even a weight gain of as little as 10 kilograms over the weight a woman had at age eighteen leads to an increased risk of death in midlife. Now I know that most of the guys reading this will immediately say, "Hey! I don't ever plan on becoming a fat nurse, so who cares?" But that would be a very foolish thing to say, guys, because not only do you not know what the future may hold—after all, as part of a midlife crisis you may very well go back to school and become a nurse one day—but more to the point, I see no reason to believe that similar results would not apply to nonnursing men as well.

Heart disease aside, excess weight is correlated with a higher risk of many other diseases, especially

- Type II diabetes
- high blood pressure
- osteoarthritis
- gallstones
- some types of cancer

Being overweight can aggravate already established conditions such as

- gastroesophageal reflux disease
- back pain
- sleep apnea

And being overweight also plays a key role in depression and poor self-image.

But, you may wonder as you try to see your toes this evening, just how are you supposed to figure out if you've got a problem with weight? As usual, this is not an easy answer. The experts always talk about BMI, or Body Mass Index, a number derived by dividing your body weight in kilograms by your height in metres squared. Anything over 25 is now potential trouble country, they say, and over 30 means that you should be reluctant to take your shirt off in public. A study found that for every 1 per cent increase in BMI above the healthy lower range, there was a corresponding increase of 10 per cent mortality from all causes in young and middle-aged men. Perhaps an easier way to gauge weight, however, is to look at those commonly available weight-and-height charts and see where you fit, or don't, as the case may be. Still another way is to look in the mirror. If the guy you see staring back at you is not the guy you would like to see—if the guy looking back at you looks much more like Jackie Gleason than like Jackie Chan—then it's probably time to shed a few pounds. By the way, if like me, you tried to do your BMI calculation and you came up with something like 658, don't panic. That's purely a tribute to your high school math teacher.

There are a couple of caveats to all that, however. First, as we have all seen, many very heavy people live to a ripe old age. How do they do it? Well, most of them are very fortunate souls, blessed with great genes and even better luck. But clearly there are also a lot of other fat people who are not genetically protected, and who also manage to live well and long. So how do these folks manage it? Because they are fit. Some of you may find this hard to imagine, but you can be fat and still fit. And people who are fit and fat do all right. In fact, statistics from the Cooper Institute for Aerobics Research in Texas show that overweight men who are fit do not have any increased risk of dying from a heart attack compared to their thinner brothers, although thin men who are not fit, do. The good news is, then, that if you are fit, you probably don't have to always maintain your ideal weight. Living within the vicinity of your ideal weight is probably good enough, and even living within a commuting suburb of the ideal is probably OK, too. But you have to be fit!

Second, it's not only how much you weigh that matters but where you put pounds on as well. Thus, someone who carries excess weight around the middle (in the classic apple shape) rather than on the hips (in the classic pear shape) seems to be in a heap more trouble than his Bartlettian bro. Weight around the middle is linked to a higher risk of insulin resistance, which is in turn related to a much higher risk of heart disease, stroke, and the whole enchilada that comes with Type II diabetes. In fact, weight around the middle may be an even better predictor of eventual mortality than is overall weight. And the more of an apple you are, the higher your risk.

Now clearly, some of the weight we carry and where we carry it is beyond our control, a product of our genes. Thus, a study from Toronto showed that although your lifestyle may determine that you end up looking like a Macintosh apple, your genes might determine whether you become a big Mac or a small Mac, and those of us who are small Macs are less likely to develop obesity-related problems than are our Fuji-wannabe brothers. Overall, the experts say, from 20 to 40 per cent of obesity is determined by your genes. But the other side of that fat coin is that 60 to 80 per cent of your excess weight is probably under your control, and it's those extra pounds that you want to attack.

So what should you do? Well, the bottom line, especially as it sags nearer and nearer to the ground, is this: if you are too big for your height, there are only two things you can do. One is to grow taller. The second is to try to lose some weight.

And there are only two ways to do that too. Do more. And eat less. Thank you very much, and you can mail the Nobel Prize to my home because I don't really ever want to visit Stockholm. Too many dour professors in too many Volvos and Saabs.

Why do more? Because the more you do, the lighter you should get, assuming, of course, you don't compensate for the extra work by eating more. But also, the more you work, the more fit you will get, and in the end, I think that being fit is far more important than weighing less.

Doing more involves learning to be more active in your daily routine and starting to do regular exercise. As to which exercise is best, any exercise that raises caloric output without at the same time increasing the urge to eat more will do (see the next section, on exercise).

Doing more is not usually enough, though. You have to learn to eat less too. But how, I hear you crying, do you get yourself to eat less? That one is clearly not easy, as the multimillion-dollar weight-loss industry can attest. Alas, despite scientists' frantic push to satisfy one of Western society's most urgent needs—to find a tiny pill that taken once a day, or even better, once a month, would allow us to have our cake and eat it too (and most of us would eat the entire cake if we could)—for now, I'm afraid, there is no miracle diet pill on the horizon. Every weight-loss pill that has come along has resulted in rare but potential health risks that far outweighed the potential benefits for anyone not seriously overweight. Although there is a host of new weight-loss miracle pills in the pipeline to take the place of those that have been removed from the market, it will be years, I think, before we can be certain that any new product does not have serious deleterious effects on health over the long term.

So for now, willpower and dieting remain the best answers for most of us. Which diet, you ask. For the two or three weeks most of us need to lose a few pounds and get a head start on learning to eat better, I think it really doesn't matter. So long as you keep a lid on your fat intake, and so long as you don't go out and replace those fatty foods with a ton of sugar and refined carbohydrates (a calorie, after all, is still a calorie), there is absolutely no proof that any sensible diet—from Pritikin to Scarsdale to The Zone to Styrofoam chips and salsa (actually, that last one may not be all that sensible)—has any better track record at helping you keep the excess weight off than do the many others you will run across.

I also suggest that you never stop trying to lose weight, if that is your goal. Don't be afraid to try dieting from time to time. You can succeed. Lots of people have. Yo-yo dieting is unlikely to be bad for your health, and losing some weight even temporarily is probably better for you than just accepting the excess poundage and doing nothing about it.

There is at least one potential drawback to dieting, however, one that every dieter will recognize, I'm sure. According to a British study, dieters use up so much brain power thinking about food that their memory capacity shrinks, and the constant focus on food makes it difficult to work. Maybe that's why it took me seven years to write this book.

Once you get to a reasonable weight, it's very important to keep eating sensibly, with an emphasis on more fruits, veggies, fibre, legumes, and grains, and to eat much less meat and fewer prepared foods. A study in the *American Journal of Public Health* found that people who eat meat seven times a week tend to gain weight, while those who eat nineteen servings of veggies a week are more likely to lose weight. The authors concluded that cutting meat to less than three servings per week might work to decrease the amount of abdominal weight most of us put on as we age. It would also reduce our enjoyment of life by 30 per cent, but hey, at least we would live longer.

Finally, I am going to end this section with a bit of a downer, I'm afraid. A study from Rockefeller University showed that the body adjusts its metabolic rate to maintain weight, so when you lose weight, your body starts to burn calories more slowly. In other words, when you cut your caloric intake, you need either to eat even less or to burn even more calories in order to lose weight. That is why, as everyone who has ever tried to lose those last five or ten pounds knows, it gets harder and harder to lose weight from dieting the closer you get to your goal.

There's also this bit of bad news: even if you work hard at trying to lose weight, it may still not be enough because according to a very depressing study, even men who run a fair amount still gain weight and spread around the middle as they hit middle age. What that means, guys, is that no matter how hard you work at staying slim, as you grow older, you must continue to increase the amount of exercise you do just to stay at the same weight. In other words, unless we work increasingly harder at eating less and exercising more, all of us middle-aged guys may be doomed by our genes and hormones to get fatter and fatter.

EXERCISE

Too many of us are too sedentary. A U.S. survey found, for example, that by age sixty-five, the average North American will have spent the equivalent of nine years in front of the tube, and that survey was done even before *Seinfeld* reruns went into syndication. Even by cheating and defining golfing and gardening as exercise, statistics from the Centers for Disease Control in Atlanta reveal that one-quarter of American adults do no physical exercise at all year-round.

And Americans are not alone in their sloth. A report prepared for the Heart and Stroke Foundation of Canada found that 35 per cent of Canadians are "essentially inactive," meaning that inactivity has now officially replaced constitution-kvetching as Canada's national sport.

What benefits can regular exercise offer? For one thing, it extends life, which is not a bad thing for most of us. Regular exercise also lowers the risk of many diseases, including:

- heart disease
- stroke
- several cancers, among them cancer of the colon and breast
- gallstones
- osteoporosis
- Type II diabetes
- Alzheimer's disease

Exercise also leads to:

- better weight control
- loss of fat
- replacement of fat with muscle
- better immunity
- fewer days off work
- less pain and inflammation
- better stress management
- lower blood pressure
- higher levels of HDL
- less deterioration in hearing and sight
- better memory
- increased creativity
- better quality and quantity of sleep
- enhanced alertness

In support of that last claim, a study from Manchester University concluded that a group of "super-fit" seventy-year-olds was just as alert as those twenty years their junior. Jogging, this study claims, is better for the brain than are crossword puzzles, although who has ever proved that crossword puzzles are good for the brain? What part of the brain is helped, I wonder, by knowing that an esme is a medieval serf, or that a tor is some kind of hill?

Although exercise has not been shown to alleviate depression, it has been shown to elevate mood and lead to a subsequent increased bout of energy.

Of more importance to many of you, exercise may help your brain and your sex life. Dr. Rodney Swain from the University of Wisconsin in Milwaukee found that rats that enjoyed running—that is, rats that were not forced to run but that did so anyway (although to be honest, I still can't picture a jogging rat)—grew new blood vessels in the brain. And they grew those blood vessels within three days of starting to run. This may help explain why regular exercise seems to protect against Alzheimer's disease and the loss of cognitive functions. As to what exercise can do for your sex life, one researcher has claimed that exercise is a "sure fire way to reawaken your sexual spirit," and you know, until I read that, I had absolutely no inkling that I even had a sexual spirit, something that made me wish that I had spent more time on my spiritual nature in my younger years.

But before you suddenly start rushing around your bedroom tonight trying to resurrect your newly discovered sexual spirit—and, one hopes, your sleeping spouse too—remember this important caveat. If you have spent your entire life being sedentary, you should be cautious about suddenly pumping your heart vigorously. As I've already noted, it can be fatal for a sedentary middle-aged male to suddenly begin exercising. So check with your doctor before embarking on an exercise program. But don't just call her on the phone. Why don't you walk to her office instead?

How much exercise do you need to do? Here, I'm afraid, the jury is still out and farting around. You see, in an attempt to encourage more people to do more, or even to do anything, many health experts have abandoned their decades-long exhortation to do vigorous exercise many days a week, and they are now claiming that as little as thirty minutes of extra work, involving as little activity as puttering around the garden, even taken in ten-minute hits three times a day, is enough. So now you have "exercise lite" to accompany your cholesterol-free eggs and fat-free mayonnaise.

But is exercise lite really good enough? We don't really know. On the one hand, a study of Harvard alumni found that vigorous exercise is correlated with better health, but nonvigorous exercise didn't do much for the best and brightest and most often quoted. In this study, 2000 or more calories per week was deemed to be the minimal necessary calorie expenditure to achieve any benefits. On the same hand, another study found that the more intense the exercise, the greater the improvement in blood pressure control, cholesterol levels, body fat, and HDL level.

On the ubiquitous other hand, however, a study from the Cooper Institute for Aerobics Research found a 15 per cent decline in mortality going from moderate fitness to high fitness but a 40 per cent lower mortality when going from no fitness to any fitness at all. In other words, a little pain, lots of gain.

What all this means for you, then, is that any exercise is better than none at all, but if you can do more, do more. To me, it seems that thirty minutes of vigorous activity at least five days a week is the minimum you should aim for. But perhaps even more important, you should aim to increase your calorie expenditure in your normal day-to-day activity as well. I can't believe the number of people who use an elevator to go up one flight of stairs, who never move their butts while on an escalator, who get their wife to take out the garbage, or who never walk to the park or the corner store. If you were simply to take the stairs each time instead of the elevator or walk to the store regularly instead of driving, you would probably improve your chances of living longer even more than you would by suddenly taking up jogging or power walking. But have your kids take out the garbage because taking out the garbage isn't likely to help you live longer.

A special note about weight loss, for which exercise lite probably does not cut it at all. The consensus from most studies is that the harder you work at your activity, the more likely you will be to lose weight. Thus, a hard thirty-minute run is much more beneficial for losing weight than a three-mile walk—so long as you are not on a one-way run to the pub to grab a few quick ones.

What about exercise equipment? Here I am a real conservative. I believe that the late Dr. George Sheehan, the original guru of the fitness movement in North America, had it right when he said, "All you need to get fit is to live in a two-story house, and have a poor memory." You don't need fancy step machines and treadmills to become fit. Even if you buy one of those overpriced gadgets, chances are you won't be using it after a few weeks anyway. I once saw a study claiming that most exercise bikes in the home were now used as clotheshorses, leading some wag to speculate that a smart company should market an exercise bike with the clothes hangers already attached. A recent survey found that 88 per cent of people who own exercise equipment would not buy home exercise equipment in the future. After all, how many clotheshorses does one really need?

I don't think you need to join a fitness group or a runner's claque either. All you really need is a simple program that is not costly and that can be done anywhere, alone. That is why walking or jogging every day is probably the best exercise regime for most of us. Walking gets you outside, walking can be done anywhere, walking is not swimming, walking is not linked to many injuries or hazards as long as you watch out for cars and dog poo, and walking can easily be done with a partner, adding a social benefit to the activity—but only if you like the partner.

And walking does work. In a study done on elderly men, the researchers concluded that a daily walk of two miles can significantly prolong life.

If for some reason you can't walk—if you have early arthritis of the hip or knee, for example—then a good alternative is to buy yourself a stationary bike. Just put it in front of the tube and peddle away.

So do it, guys. It's never too late to start, even for a guy who last moved his huge butt the day his team won the cup in 1979. Tell yourself it's time, get checked out by your doctor, and then just do it, man.

SLEEP

We don't get enough sleep. Why? Because sleep is like the federal budget: it's just too simple to run a deficit and pretend that you will pay it back one day.

We haven't always been that dumb. The feds used to balance their budgets, and we used to sleep when we were tired. One hundred years ago, the Better Sleep Council claims, the average North American slept 20 per cent longer than we do now. Turn-of-the-century adults, who did not have the allure of all-night, mind-blowing entertainment like *Rockford Files* reruns and *Jerry Springer*, slept about 9½ hours a night. Today 60 per cent of modern-day Americans get an average of less than 7 hours of sleep.

Sleep deprivation exerts a heavy price, both in immediate and in long-term negative effects on our health and well-being. On an immediate level:

- Fatigue from lack of sleep is a major contributor to motor vehicle accidents. According to one study of subjects' reflexes, for example, even moderate levels of fatigue produced levels of "impaired performance" similar to the performance deficit seen at a blood alcohol concentration of .05 per cent, and the researchers weren't referring to the kind of performance deficit most men usually worry about either.
- Any interruption of the normal sleep schedule for only a few hours causes people to be moodier and more anxious.
- Sleep deprivation also has a negative effect on higher brain functions such as thinking skills.
- Even three hours of sleep deprivation can lower immunity by decreasing the number of circulating "natural killer cells," those mean little Oliver Stones in your blood stream that nab any predators that dare invade your body. The good news is that a good night's sleep quickly restores those cell levels to normal.

Because memories and learning are also consolidated during sleep, any new skills you acquire are much more easily stored and recalled if that learning is followed by a proper night's sleep.

The long-term effects of poor sleep are harder to gauge, but several long-term studies have linked chronic sleep abnormalities with greater disability and poorer health outcomes, even with reduced life expectancy.

How much sleep do you need? That one's easy: enough sleep to feel rested the next day. Most people require 8 to 8½ hours of sleep per night, but many people do fine on only 6 or even fewer hours of sleep and other people need 11 hours. The most common reason for not getting enough sleep is the obvious. We simply don't get to bed on time, and even if we do, it's often not to sleep. That is sleep deprivation through choice. But there are lots of unfortunate people who have no choice, who don't get enough sleep because they just can't sleep well enough or long enough. Although there are over eighty recognized sleep disorders, they can be divided into three main types:

- an inability to fall asleep
- poor quality of sleep—that is, not sleeping soundly but tossing and turning
- early rising—that is, having no difficulty falling asleep but jolting awake several hours later, far too soon to have gotten a good night's sleep

These sleep disorders can all be caused by anxiety or stress, other medical conditions, or depression.

All the strategies discussed in Chapter 2 can work for a temporary acute inability to sleep. Far too often, however, a seemingly one-off or three-off sleepless night becomes chronic. When it does, it mimics impotence in that the more you think about it, the harder it gets to deal with. Don't let that happen to you. If a temporary sleep problem is lingering, talk to your doctor about it. Studies show that although 20 to 30 per cent of adults have some complaints of insomnia, most don't talk to their doctor about it. That is too bad, because this is one problem for which we have some pretty good strategies and aids, starting with a long wait in the doctor's office, which generally puts most insomniacs to sleep even before they can get in to see the doctor.

What about drugs? I have no hesitation in advising anyone with a case of acute insomnia to take a sleeping medication, and even several in a row during a particularly bad week, as when your kid suddenly returns home from school, at the age of thirty—to stay—with his family and three dogs. The problem with all these drugs, however, is that it is easy to become reliant on them. Never take sedatives or hypnotics for more than a few days in a row without having a long chat with your physician about what else you can do to ease your problem, such as changing the locks on your front door. It is also important to be aware that all sleeping pills, but especially the longer-acting ones, can produce sleepiness the next day and a consequent increased risk of accidents.

A quick few words about those special sleep-related problems, snoring and sleep apnea. From 50 to 80 per cent of all men snore at least part of the night. With the exception of those snorers who suffer from sleep apnea, which is about 4 to 5 per cent of all heavy snorers, the huge majority of snorers do not suffer any undue consequences from their snoring, no matter how loud it is. The same cannot be said, however, about their bedmates, whose health and sanity are often unduly affected by the incessant nightly cacophony at their side.

Snoring occurs when air moves over an obstruction or through a narrowed channel. Thus, anything that lessens muscle tone in the neck and throat and allows the tissues to collapse more can make snoring worse. Snoring is thus made worse by

- being sedentary and weak-muscled
- being older
- being obese
- having allergies
- using alcohol
- using tranquillizers or drugs with a sedating effect, such as some antihistamines
- having large tonsils and adenoids
- having a large uvula, nasal polyps, or a large tongue

The treatment of snoring starts with removing the snorer to another bedroom. This usually solves the problem instantly for the bedmate. For the snorer, it's more advisable to first attack any known contributing factor, such as minimizing the use of alcohol. Other strategies include elevating the head of the bed (the more upright you are, the less the tissues collapse, although many heavy snorers can sleep and snore just as well standing up), and using gadgets or reminders or strategies that lead to frequent changes of position, especially those that get the snorer off his back (my wife, for example, routinely kicks me during the night, and I must say that I really resent that, mostly because I don't snore).

If all else fails, you might try one of those surgical techniques to remove the uvula and shrink the tissues at the back of the throat, but be aware that the long-term consequences of these procedures have not yet been established. And finally, for women reading this, you can always try a husbandectomy.

As for sleep apnea, a recent study reports that this condition is most severe in middle-aged men. In sleep apnea, loud snoring is associated with a cessation in breathing for a period ranging from a few seconds to as long as ninety seconds on several and often many occasions a night. Several studies have linked sleep apnea to a higher risk of stroke and heart attack. Not everyone agrees with this morbid connection, however. A group of laid-back Brits—the kind of people who get excited only when a dictator is camping on their doorstep—claimed in a recent study that sleep apnea is not nearly as serious as we've been led to believe and that despite what North American experts claim, there is really only weak evidence linking sleep apnea with a higher risk of heart attack and stroke. I prefer to believe the North Americans.

Risk factors for sleep apnea include chronic loud snoring, obesity, and high blood pressure. You should suspect that you might have sleep apnea if first, a bedmate tells you that when you sleep you sound like a sputtering eighteen-wheeler trying to rev its motor, and second, if you also suffer from such sleep loss-related symptoms as

- daytime fatigue
- excessive sleepiness
- memory impairment
- a recurrent tendency to crash your car

Sleep apnea is best diagnosed in a sleep lab and not by a wife.

Treatment starts with losing weight if you happen to be overweight, and minimizing the use of alcohol and sedatives. More active therapy consists of devices worn at night that deliver a stream of air pressure to the nose and sometimes surgery.

SMOKING

A very few words about the number one health scourge. If you are a smoker and you decide to make only one change in your life to improve your chances of living long enough to witness the next millennium's first major attraction—the day the bloated Olympics implode from the weight of too many curlers, hurlers, ice dancers, rhythmic swimmers, and bureaucrats—give up smoking. I know how hard it is to do, I know how the tobacco companies have conspired to keep you addicted, I know how difficult your life is going to be for a few weeks or maybe even months, I know of the overheated claims that tobacco addiction is harder to beat than heroin addiction, but c'mon! Gimme a break! You're not a kid anymore, you have surely dealt with more difficult matters, and if you haven't then you certainly will pretty soon, and this task should be not much harder for the average man to deal with than most of the other difficult issues in life. Just give it up. It's time.

Smoking, the experts say, can kill you in twenty-four ways, and it's working on each of those killer tracks simultaneously even as you sit there reading this. What's in it for you, if you give up smoking, is that not only will you significantly reduce your risks of dying from all sorts of illnesses, such as a heart attack and many forms of cancer, but you will also lessen your chances of dying from some undignified disease such as terminal emphysema. Even better, if you stop smoking, you will also be helping all the newborns and infants and toddlers and even adults around you minimize their risks of secondhand smoke-related diseases. A recent study found, for example, that spending as little as one-half hour in a room with a smoker leads to a fall in antioxidant levels in the blood, which would eventually result in a higher risk of heart attack, stroke, and other degenerative illnesses.

Are there any secret miracle methods for quitting smoking? No. You have to want to quit, and if you want to badly enough, they will all probably work equally well.

Perhaps best of all, when you finally quit, you will also be giving the finger to those damnable tobacco honchos who got you addicted in the first place. Wouldn't you just love to be part of a major movement that put a couple of tobacco companies out of the death business one day?

STRESS

Stress is rampant. One survey found, for example, that two-thirds of Americans feel stressed out at least once a week, and that's just the over-the-top I-can't-manage-cuz-it's-all-just-wearing-me-down kind of stress. The more niggling, one-off, gee-I-hope-the-test-comes-back-normal-because-I-don't-know-what-I'm-gonna-tell-what's-his-name kind of stress is much more prevalent, but it affects you just as adversely.

Many of the negative effects of excess stress have already been mentioned, but to pull it all together and to add a few new bits, excess stress is related to:

- a higher risk of suffering a heart attack or stroke or cardiac-associated sudden death
- high blood pressure
- erectile problems
- depression and suicide
- gastroesophageal reflux
- sick-building syndrome

Stress also:

- slows healing of wounds
- impairs immunity
- impairs the blood-brain barrier
- may lead to fat around the middle, which not only is unsightly but is also a major health risk
- interrupts testosterone production (perhaps that's why my voice goes up so high when I'm stressed)
- lowers sperm counts
- impairs memory
- leaves you more open to coming down with a nasty cold

And most scary, perhaps, stress probably also affects men in subtle ways that we are not yet completely aware of. For example, when a male cichlid fish is under chronic high stress, he fails to develop the "bright, war-like colors, the extra muscles and the [ohmygawd!] fully mature sex organs" he is naturally prone to develop. Now that's scary.

What's so curious about these negative effects of stress is that a stress reaction started out as something very useful, and in its place it still is. That old fight-or-flight reaction in response to some perceived danger or threat to your well-being—a marauding bear, for example, or an apple-bearing snake—has served from the beginning as a very useful, often lifesaving response. Back on the savanna, when a tiger came around to see which one of our ancestors he would prefer for lunch, it was useful for each of those endangered beings to instantly secrete a flood of stress hormones, which in turn mobilized and jump-started his brain and other neurological and endocrine systems to get him the hell out of there, a very good thing for him and an even better one for us or else many of us wouldn't be here. Today we may not have to flee from tigers, but their legacy remains. Our modern-day ersatz hero, faced with the equivalent of a tiger—another driver cutting him off, for example, or a spouse who wants to paint the house again when it was last done only twelve years ago—is still able to mount an instant put-em-up-or-I'm-outta-here stress response and jump-start his biochemical and neurological systems.

Now each individual stress reaction is unlikely to do much harm, assuming, that is, that it doesn't kill you instantly, because a stressful event can indeed sometimes result in sudden cardiac death. For example, managers who fire someone double their risk of suffering a heart attack for the week after they sack the employee.

For most of us, however, stress is more likely to kill us slowly. Repeated pulses of stress hormone wear down our bodies and lead to all those deleterious effects that were mentioned earlier.

Some of us are more at risk than others, however. Take for example, a study that found that stressed-out Finnish men who don't ski-jump have much higher rates of coronary heart disease than those who do because of the constant ribbing the former face from the rest of the nation. Just kidding, of course, because there are no Finns who don't ski-jump. What this study really concluded is that some Finnish men were more likely to react to stress by developing coronary heart disease than were other Finnish men.

But why do some men react to stress worse than others? No one knows, although we do know that genetics and early environment are important factors. For example, a study from McGill University has shown that rats that are handled in infancy seem to be better adjusted—they explore more—than rats that were not handled as infants. Some of us are just programmed, it seems, either through our genes or as a result of our early development, to handle stress more poorly than others.

Our social and economic environment is also very important. A recent Centers for Disease Control report from the U.S. found that the lowest rates of mental stress were found in employed, educated, middle-class, middle-aged Americans, although curiously the overall lowest rates were reported by sixty-five-year-old men living in South Dakota. (That's still not enough reason to move to Pierre, though.)

Now I realize that by middle age all of you have developed certain techniques to help you deal with your stress load. Some men pray, some men pay, some men play, many golf, some yell, some run, some smoke, some drink, and many men do several or all of the preceding and then some. If these tactics work for you, by all means continue to use them (all except smoking and excess drinking, of course, and maybe golf too). If, however, you are not doing well, if you are feeling too stressed, if you are beginning to lose it or to burn out, if you or those who care for you perceive that you are not handling things with your usual aplomb, then it's time to do something before the stress gets you.

- You can start by exercising regularly, something most experts push.
- Also, you can buy any one of a host of books or visual aids that can teach you how to relax, like my favourite, *The Relaxation Response* by Herbert Benson, MD.
- If you're one of those men who erupts easily, you should also work on anger control. As already noted, a sudden burst of anger can raise the risk of heart attack for up to two hours afterwards. So rather than blowing up the next time you argue, let her win. Smile over your canned tuna as your dog is contentedly digesting the steak he grabbed from your kitchen counter. It's not worth getting upset about such trivial matters. As it happens, this same study found that positive emotions such as feeling happy were associated with a lower risk of cardiac ischemia. So go one better: give the dog another steak. Ask your wife if she would like to go to a movie with (her words) the biggest moron on the block. You'll live longer for it. And as a bonus, if you reduce your anger, your sex life might improve too. A report from Exeter University in England claims that bad drivers—those prone to road rage—are terrible lovers. Stop honking, start boinking.
- You might also think of getting married, but only if you're not

already hitched, because bigamy is, I believe, quite stressful. Lots of studies show that marriage is good for your stress level.

- Learn to laugh more. Psychologists at the University of Akron in Ohio asked thirty-three men and women to compare their sense of humour with that of a sibling who had died, and most said they laughed more than their sibs ever had. Well, they certainly laughed more after the sib died, didn't they?

- You might also try to get some friends, hard as that may be for some of you guys to do, because men who have no social and emotional support are more than twice as likely to die after a heart attack than those with a caring family and friends. You have to pick the right family and friends, though, because conflict with close family members has been shown to set off stress reactions in heart disease patients, and if in them, why not in you too?

- You might also think of enrolling yourself in some classes because people without a high school education are twice as likely to have a heart attack triggered by anger as people who have at least some college education.

- You should also get a pet. Studies show that caring for pets lowers stress levels, and a study from the University of Buffalo Medical School found that in times of high stress, even a supportive partner can't get your blood pressure and heart rate down as much as a pet can, although I strongly recommend starting with a bird or a worm, not a Doberman or a pit bull.

- Here's a key one: try to become more optimistic, or at the very least stop being such a pessimist. A six-year-long Finnish study found that middle-aged men who feel hopeless about the future and about their chances of attaining their goals are far more likely to die early from coronary heart disease, accidents, and violent deaths than are equally healthy but more hopeful men. So stop being so pessimistic and think positively instead. Your son will move out one day. Taxes will eventually fall. And I will become the next Pope.

- But remember: you can't just fake optimism and good vibes. According to a British researcher, those people who constantly have to pretend to be in a good mood, such as those folks who greet you when you walk into the Gap or Wal-Mart, are more likely to develop stress-related diseases such as high blood pressure and heart disease than other people, due to the constant strain of faking a good mood. So don't have a nice day, OK?

- You might also start worrying about different things from the ones that usually consume you. A study in *Circulation* found that worries about social conditions correlated most closely with negative effects on the heart. So no more Mr. Nice Guy. It's bad for your heart. Feel good about it the next time you coldly pass a beggar or a busker asking for a handout. A cold heart is a healthy heart, and besides, maybe if we stop supporting them, all those terrible penny-whistling buskers will disappear.

- If none of that is working, however, you simply have to learn to become less of a male. That does not mean that you have to get one of those operations or take some of those hormones, but it does mean that you have to learn to reach out for help, a very unmacho thing to do. For example, in a letter to the *Lancet*, researchers from Gotland, Sweden, summed up their experience with depressed men as follows: "Men are incapable of asking for help or showing weakness."

- Now I don't want to get too touchy-feely here and I certainly don't mean that you have to put your arm around your best buddy's shoulder tonight and stare into his eyes and murmur, "John, there's something I've been meaning to tell you," mainly because John will panic, spill his beer, and fly right out of there. What I do mean is that if stress is getting the best of you, you simply have to get up the guts to talk to someone about it, preferably a professional, and bartenders and hookers are not the kind of professionals I mean. If you don't get some help, you run the great risk of getting those stress-related diseases mentioned earlier or of harming yourself by burning out (or if you're an American postal worker, harming others), or worse, of starting to rely on inappropriate stress-relief strategies, like, for example, drinking too much or golfing excessively, a terrible remedy for stress in that it invariably increases marital strife.

CHAPTER 8

My Way

Health is a state of complete physical, mental and social well-being,
not merely the absence of disease or infirmity.

—Constitution of the World Health Organization

It's not that I'm afraid to die.
I just don't want to be there when it happens.

—Woody Allen, *Death (A Play)*

So there you have it, guys. Just about all you really need to know about
what you are going through or are about to go through, and most
important, what you can still do to make your later years happier and
healthier. Sadly, however, no matter how well armed you are with all
the appropriate information and no matter how hard you try to follow
my sage advice, I'm afraid that I have some bad news: you are not going
to live forever. What is perhaps saddest is that even if you don't smoke
(or at least, if you want to be head of state one day, you don't inhale);
you scrupulously minimize your exposure to all toxins, even so far as
to avoid wearing leather shoes or sitting on leather couches just to be
100 per cent certain that you don't come down with Mad Cow Disease;
you have a great social support system, since you work hard at being a
good spouse and worker and parent and member of your community;
you never go out in the sun without a hat on and without lathering on
the sunscreen; you practise safe sex even when you're alone because
hey, these days you never can tell (just ask George Michael); you eat all
the veggies placed in front of you even if they've been prepared in the

British manner (boiled and blanched and then stored for three weeks before being reheated and served cold two hours later); you exercise diligently; and you meditate twice a day, you may still be doomed to see that lazy sloth next door whose idea of a healthy meal is anything deep-fried and accompanied by chips, and who never moves his butt except to get in the car to buy more smokes and beer, live a disease-free life while you may go on to develop dozens of health problems, not the least of which is terminal envy of that Billy Bob Bubba next door. There really is no justice when it comes to health and well-being, and you will probably only kill yourself waiting for it or expecting it, because to a greater extent than we want to believe, we are captive to our early environment and especially to our genes.

C'est la vie, I'm afraid. Our genes are simply too much with us, and they play a huge role in determining how long and how well we live, or as the authors of a study that tried to determine why some ants live longer than other ants concluded, "Mortality is largely prey to count-less processes that follow an evolutionary dictate." And as for ants, so for ant squishers. Thus, according to a study in the *Lancet*, siblings of individuals over one hundred years old are much more likely to live to ninety than people whose siblings died younger.

Happily, however, we can modify some of the effects our genes exert, and that's what you should always aim to do—work on the lifestyle factors that are known to affect health and well-being, especially the ones that you feel are worth working on. Everything I've written has been geared to urging you to do just that.

When you've had enough of doing "just that," however, it's equally important to lean back, stop feeling guilty about what you have still not gotten around to doing and may in fact never get around to doing, and relax. Relax and enjoy these best years of your life before the next stage of your all-too-brief sojourn in this mortal realm catches up to you. Maximizing happiness is what it's all about.

While you're still in the happy bloom of middle age, though, you are still in need of some regular maintenance. And because you are a child of an era in which the high priests are high-priced consultants and experts, you will also be much less anxious about your fleeting moments in the sun if some consultant—and happily for you, I am quite prepared to be that guru, and the only charge I will levy is the price of this book—comes up with some rules and homilies to help keep you happy.

So read on, dear reader, about what you need to do to keep your perch on top as long as your fingernails hold out. Be warned, though, that as soon as the really serious bits are out of the way, most of the rest of these suggestions are not the usual bits of advice you will find in books on prevention of illness (not even in the chapter I dedicated to that subject). Rather, they are gleanings from my wide reading that might interest you.

THE SERIOUS STUFF

As already mentioned, I am a cynical realist. Therefore, I know that despite my pleading and exhortations, most of you will not do too much of what I have advised you to do. Instead, you will pick one of the readily available excuses that come in a handy boxed set available from Wal-Mart—you're too old, it's too hard, there's not enough time, you're allergic to exercise, you don't have the right clothes, you don't want to outlive your kids—and wave it at anyone, especially your wife, who tries to get you to follow a more healthy lifestyle. I also know that to augment that choice, you will begin to rely much more on doctors to get you through the inevitable health valleys you waddle into. Most middle-aged men seem to labour under the false impression that all they have to do to keep their health together or to reassemble it when it breaks down temporarily (they hope) is to get an annual physical examination, which will undoubtedly detect the few potentially life-threatening diseases they are prone to at a stage when those problems are still treatable, and some medications to fix whatever abnormalities are detected. As if.

An Annual Physical Examination Is about As Valuable
As a Look into One of The Spice Girls' Minds
I hate to prick your balloon, guys, but annual physical examinations for middle-aged gents are overrated. I don't meant to imply that men especially like to have an annual physical. ("You really ought to visit this new doctor I've just been to. Man, there is nothing quite like the feeling this guy gives you when he tells you to turn your head and cough.") It's that men tend to think that an annual physical is an insurance policy against sudden death. Wrong. Although getting an annual full physical examination that turns out to be normal will no doubt lower your anxiety level and help you sleep better (it will certainly help

your doctor sleep better, given the fees that annual physical exams demand), there is absolutely no proof that in healthy individuals annual complete physical exams save lives. Nor is an annual physical exam likely to detect important hidden medical problems. Why? Because during midlife, I'm afraid, most of us get symptoms when we get sick, and it's very rare for a routine physical exam to detect a cancer, for example, or another metabolic abnormality, in a middle-aged man before the disease has betrayed its presence with symptoms that the patient ought to have noticed.

That is not to say that doctors don't detect abnormalities when they do routine physicals. They find lots of them, but most of those abnormalities are of no real importance. They are not harbingers of life-limiting disease, and you really didn't need to know they were there. Once an abnormality is picked up, however, the doctor often feels obligated, from the sudden anxiety evident in the patient's demeanour, to do some tests "just to be sure" there's nothing wrong ("I think we should do a CT scan, George, just to be sure this is a real paper cut"). Not only do medical tests invariably produce even greater anxiety, they often also carry a small degree of risk—even a blood test can result in a blood clot, and there is a very tiny potential risk of infection.

So the next time you're tempted to go for a physical examination even though your health has been excellent, just remember this old homily you can needlepoint onto something to hang on your bedroom wall: the more doctors poke, the more they find. The more they find, the more they test. The more they test, the more they find.

Having condemned annual physical exams, I do not want to give you the idea that all routine examinations are a waste of time. On the contrary, some routine exams are vital. Most important, those men who have health problems or who have particular health risks—if you have a family history of premature death from heart disease, for example, or if you have had an abnormal blood glucose test (see Chapter 5) —should definitely get regular checkups. Your special risks and the state of your health determine how often and for what you need to be examined.

But even if you have no health risks, you should still have some partial exams regularly. At the very least:

- You need to get your skin examined for skin cancer regularly—by a doctor, not your wife—because I just don't believe that any of us does a good enough job of skin self-examination. Although no one really knows how often you should have your skin pored over by a health professional, I think once a year is about right for most of us aging ex-sun gods. This is especially important if you are at high risk for malignant melanoma. Who is at high risk? Anyone who has had lots of sun exposure or previous skin cancers, has fair skin, is redheaded, or has a history of bad sunburns in childhood and adolescence.

- You should have your blood pressure taken once a year, and not just by those shopping-centre machines but by a real, live, honest-to-goodness human.
- You might also want to have your prostate palpated regularly. Perhaps I should rephrase that and say that you should have your prostate palpated regularly—probably once a year—whether you want to or not.

You also need to get some medical tests on a regular basis. Unfortunately, the number crunchers and health bureaucrats have turned routine screening into a political minefield, and some of these tests are not covered by some medical plans, so you may need to reach into your own huge resources and pay for some of these yourselves.

- As a healthy midlife man, you should get your cholesterol profile (see Chapter 5) done at least once.

Other tests that you should have regularly include:

- PSA (see Chapter 4)
- blood glucose (see Chapter 5)
- stool test for occult blood
- perhaps a sigmoidoscopy (or colonoscopy)

I must make special note here of the last two tests.

A stool test for occult blood is a test generally honoured in the breach. This is a big mistake. Colorectal cancer is the third leading cause of cancer deaths in men. Although genetics plays a strong role in the risk for colon cancer—Ashkenazi Jews, for example, as well as first-degree relatives of anyone who has had colon cancer at a young age (before fifty) are at much higher risk than the general population—the most important risk factors seem to be age and diet. The longer you live, the less fibre you eat, and the less balanced your diet, the more likely you are to rue your bowel. Regular exercise also seems to lower the risk of colon cancer.

As to what you can do to prevent colon cancer, no surprises there—the best thing to do is to follow a well-balanced diet with lots of fibre and get plenty of exercise.

Perhaps the best news, though, is that most colon cancers can be apprehended as precancerous polyps when they are often easily surgically removed. Snipping the polyp usually prevents it from turning into a cancer.

Currently, the best large-scale screening test for colon cancer is the stool test for occult blood, in which the patient collects three samples of stool and submits them (on a special card, to be sure, and with delicacy) to the lab, where they are checked for microscopic amounts of blood, which is shed by polyps and cancers.

The benefits of this test are enormous: it is easy, portable (although I do think this is better done at home), private (not necessarily if you live with a teenager), and cheap. So why don't we do more of this test? Because patients hate doing it. This is really too bad because several studies have shown that in large populations, annual screening with stool tests for occult blood saves lives. So the best advice is this, guys: put a leash on your dignity. Sit yourself down with a good read (such as this book), and just do it. Three times.

The other test that is often recommended as a routine screen for colon cancer every five years or so is a sigmoidoscopy or (colonoscopy), in which you lie on the table in a very undignified manner while a doctor shoves a tube up where the sun will never shine (a gastroenterologist friend of mine who does a lot of these procedures describes them as "a case of one arsehole looking up another arsehole"). In a sigmoidoscopy, the tube goes only (I use the word "only" simply in a comparative sense, of course) part way through the large bowel, while in a colonoscopy the doctor goes for the Whopper—all the way into the right side of the colon. Been there and had that done, and all I can say is that my gastroenterologist friend is absolutely dead on.

"Be Careful about Reading Health Books.
You Might Die of a Misprint"—Mark Twain
In midlife, some men begin to visit the doctor whenever they feel ill, because unfortunately, midlife is when those men begin to see death's

visage staring back at them in every itch or cough or red blotch that pops up. This is when a wife becomes indispensable, because a wife is the one person who will invariably tell you the only two words you really need to hear during these panic attacks: "Grow up."

If a wife doesn't do it for you, though, let me warn you about beginning to rely on your doctor to alleviate your concerns about every new symptom or every time you feel ill. The doctor is not a magician. She does not have other-worldly diagnostic skills (a study has estimated that nearly 50 per cent of visits to the doctor end without a diagnosis that can be confirmed), and she doesn't possess a grab bag of miracle potions. You may have misplaced it over the years, but most of you were born with a modicum of good sense. Find it and use it. Instead of your doctor, rely more on the time-tested remedy of "tincture of time," and you'll probably do just as well, often even better.

Unfortunately, there is no cut-and-dried set of rules to tell you when a visit to the doctor is necessary, and everyone has a story about a "Poor Joe. Didn't see the doctor with his four-day cough and now he has pneumonia." We should all feel sorry for Poor Joe, of course, but the truth is that it's very unlikely Poor Joe's doctor could have prevented his pneumonia even if Poor Joe had been sitting in the doctor's office all during his illness, a practice many patients would love to be able to follow, by the way. So for all the Poor Joes out there, remember this: most pneumonias are not preventable with our current array of medications, and in most circumstances (absence of high fever, chest pain, and shortness of breath), waiting a few days with a cough (or headache or sore throat or muscle ache or . . .) is not likely to make any difference in the outcome.

"But," some of you are no doubt sputtering, "even if it doesn't do us any good to see the doctor quickly with our symptoms, surely it can't do us any harm." Poor naïve babies. First, think back to that old needlepoint homily from a few paragraphs ago. But even more important, doctors make mistakes. A Harris poll in the U.S. found that 42 per cent of respondents claim that they or a friend or a relative have experienced a "medical mistake." Fortunately, most of those errors were probably minor and didn't involve loss of life (although I am not sure how they would have gone about trying to poll those who were actually killed by medical mistakes), but even minor errors can be uncomfortable or lead to further problems.

If You Do Visit the Doctor, Ask Why, Why, Why

You can, though, minimize your risks of ending up as a medical statistic if you become more like the patients I am used to seeing. No, I don't mean you have to turn into a converted ex-hippy who now drives a Volvo station wagon instead of a painted-on Beetle and who is more interested in selling the doctor stock tips than hashish (never inhaled, by the way). Rather, what I mean is that you need to be a lot more assertive and skeptical in your doctor's office. Thus, when you visit your family doc, always make sure to ask lots of questions and always challenge him to answer your concerns. Not only do you deserve the answers—after all, one way or the other you are paying for the information—but the right answer might even save your life one day.

So when you leave a doctor's office, the bare minimum you should know is the answer to these questions:

- What do I have? (Oh, it's a virus.)
- What else could it be? (You don't think it's Ebola, do you? I know I haven't been to Africa, but hey, I did go to the zoo once when I was a kid.)
- When should I expect to be better? (Should I tell my boss I won't be back till 2000? [For unionized workers, 2003.])
- What should I do if I am not better in that time? (What if I get the millennium bug on top of this?)
- What can I do to make myself better? (Rest at home? Have more sex?)
- Should I contact you again? (Why are you sneering, doc?)

If you receive a prescription, here are a few more things you should know:

- What is this drug?
- Why this drug?
- How safe is it?
- Are there any alternative medications?
- How do I take it?
- Anything I should avoid while I'm on it?
- Anything it interacts with?

If you are sent for tests, some other questions you need to have answered are:

- Why do I need this test?
- Is it safe—what are the risks?
- How accurate is it?
- When will you have the results?
- Can I get the results over the phone? This is a pet peeve of mine. With certain exceptions—the HIV test is the most obvious example— I believe that most test results can be given over the phone, although for various reasons—fees, ease on the staff, concern about how the patient will take the result—many doctors seem to prefer to give test results in a face-to-face meeting. Given that most tests are done for routine reasons, either as screening tests or to rule out the possibility of certain abnormalities, most test results are normal. It seems to me to be an unbelievable waste of time, effort, and money to have someone come back to the office to hear that "your cholesterol level [or throat culture or Pap smear] was normal. Next."

Now on first thought, you might think that the answers to all the questions I listed would take the doctor about a year to dispense. As a long-time family physician, however, I can tell you that most of us have learned to speak so fast that we go through this checklist in only a few minutes, and those few minutes are a good investment in preventing needless extra visits to the office.

When It Comes to Drugs: Just Say No (More Often)
We live in a culture and an era that demands chemical answers for every symptom or illness—a pill for every ill, "a med for my head else I'm dead"—and too many doctors are only too keen to feed our habit. Happily, most of the time, the medications you get from your doctor or take on your own are helpful. But as that Harris poll I referred to earlier also found, at least 28 per cent of patients know they have been subjected to a drug error, and if you factor in all those patients who have no clue that the drug they were taking caused their hair to turn green or their feet to smell like ripe cheese (more than usually, that is), that rate of drug error is probably much higher.

There are many ways to be harmed by drugs. You can, of course, simply receive the wrong medication for your condition, or the wrong dose. But what may surprise you is that even the right drug at the proper dose can harm you. Adverse drug reactions stem from the *proper* use of drugs—no mistakes were made when the drugs were used, and the drugs were only doing what they were supposed to do. Adverse drug reactions are caused by side effects that occur at normal doses, interactions with other drugs, an exaggerated response in an individual to a normal dose of a drug, or an allergic or idiosyncratic reaction.

Unfortunately, adverse drug reactions are very common. A study in the *Journal of the American Medical Association* estimated that up to 30 per cent of hospitalized patients are subject to an adverse drug reaction, while another study in the same journal claimed that adverse drug reactions may account for 100,000 deaths a year in the U.S. There is no reason to believe it's any different anywhere else.

So if they can be so dangerous, why do doctors give out so many drugs? Because you want them, and it's far easier for a doctor to give you what you want than it is to spend the extra time and effort convincing you that medication is not the answer to your problem; because doctors want to help and the quickest salvation comes from a salve or a pill; and because doctors and the public tend to ignore the potential harmful consequences of medication while focussing only on the benefits. It's also savvy in this era of malpractice suits to give something, anything, even if the condition doesn't warrant it. Thus, patients who expect a drug are between three and ten times as likely to get one as those who don't expect one. This one really is a no-brainer: if you want to minimize your risk of getting sick from a drug, don't smell like you're looking for meds when you go into your doctor's office.

There are certain groups of drugs that are especially likely to be abused.

First, of course, are antibiotics. Many, perhaps even most, antibiotic prescriptions are unnecessary, especially those dispensed for upper respiratory infections, which are most often caused by viruses and thus are not amenable to the usual battery of bug killers. Worse, the more antibiotics we give out, the faster those little bacteria develop resistance to them. This problem of bacterial resistance to multiple drugs is now so severe that several experts have warned that we may be on the brink of an era in which we will not be able to treat some of the common infections that used to kill us before antibiotics came along. So don't use antibiotics when you don't have to.

Unfortunately, you shouldn't expect your doctor to help you much on this one. Doctors are still, I'm afraid, dispensing antibiotics far too often and for the wrong reasons, and no one really knows how to stop them. Or as a headline from an editorial in the *Lancet* a while back asked: "What will it take to stop physicians from prescribing anti-biotics in acute bronchitis?" Smarter patients for a start.

A second class of drugs you need to be wary of are nonsteroidal anti-inflammatory drugs, such as ASA and ibuprofen, especially since many of them are available over the counter. These are all excellent medications for relief of both pain and inflammation. They have also been touted as being able to prevent colon polyps and Alzheimer's disease. But regular use of all nonsteroidal anti-inflammatory drugs can cause stomach ulcers, which not only bleed and sometimes hemorrhage but which can also perforate—unfortunately, they can suddenly appear as life-threatening crises without any previous warning signs. Non-steroidal anti-inflammatories can interact with many other medications, and they can also raise blood pressure, especially for someone who is already on blood pressure-lowering medication.

One of the other important problems associated with the use of all painkillers, including nonsteroidal anti-inflammatories, when they are used for the treatment of headaches, especially migraines, is the potential for a sort of addiction. It's not that the person with the chronic headaches becomes addicted so much as his body becomes addicted, so when he decides not to use the medication, the body signals its displeasure by producing—you guessed it—a headache. This is known as a rebound phenomenon, and it's very common in people who have used analgesics regularly for several years.

If you decide to take a drug, here are a few warnings. First, always take the smallest dose of the weakest medication for the least amount of time that will do the trick. If, however, you get a prescription for antibiotics, always take the full amount.

Second, this may sound like your mother talking, but remember, a drug only works if you take it. Sit up straight, by the way. And wipe that smile off your face, midlife man. What I mean is that if you want to get your cholesterol levels down, the cholesterol-lowering medication won't work if it stays in your medicine cabinet.

And here's what may seem like an odd bit of advice: if you are taking a drug, you should probably avoid grapefruit. Grapefruit juice removes large amounts of a certain enzyme from the lining of the small intestine. This enzyme is very important in breaking down some commonly used drugs, such as calcium channel blockers, estro-gens, caffeine, theophyllin, and several others as they are absorbed into the body. Thus, more of the drug is absorbed and this increased absorption can in turn lead to dangerously high blood levels of that medication.

Finally, I'll end this serious section with a last important piece of health advice that I couldn't fit anywhere else in this text: do testicular self-examination, or TSE, regularly. "What do I do?" I hear some of you lesser lights asking. Easy, man. All you gotta do is roll your own.

NOW FOR THE LESS SERIOUS BITS

Get Married

Many studies have shown that married men outlive their single counterparts, often by several years. Why? It may simply be that healthier people tend to get married in the first place, but more likely it's because marriage lessens stress (see Chapter 1) and because married men tend to lead healthier lifestyles, mostly, of course, because we're forced to.

And for those cynics—mostly married men—who say that a married man doesn't really live any longer, he just feels as if he's never going to be allowed to die, the consensus is that marriage does lead to better health. A British report concluded that not only do married people live longer, they also suffer lower rates of cancer and heart disease, as well as less stress and mental illness than do both single people and cohabiters, those who live together but who haven't been dragooned into tying the knot.

If, however, you feel that an extra few years of life gained at the expense of being nagged to "put out that cigarette, put down that glass of wine, put away those five salami sandwiches" is not reason enough to get hitched, here's something else that might induce you to march up the aisle. According to a report from the Population Association of America, marriage increases wealth. At least that's what the experts who did this study say, although I'm not sure what the actual men in the marriages would say.

So if you haven't already done so, get married. Besides, by fifty, don't you think it's finally time you got your mother off your back? Let a wife deal with her. She will know how to do it better and with less stress.

Wash Your Hands Constantly

Less than half of us wash our hands after going to the washroom, and the experts claim that this is unhealthy, although I have always wondered why washing your hands is such an important thing for men to do. I mean, what kind of bacteria lurk on your zipper anyway? That aside, washing your hands often, even when not visiting the washroom regularly, is one of the easiest ways to minimize your risk of picking up and passing on infections, and in this era where the dreaded flesh-eating strep is lurking in who-knows-what spots to get you and your kin, you would be well advised to wash your hands. Often.

You should also make sure that anyone taking care of you when you're sick washes his or her hands often. A study of health care workers found that many of them do not wash their hands when examining a new patient, even though hand washing is widely viewed as vital—perhaps even as the single most important, and certainly the simplest, procedure—in preventing the spread of infection. Happily, this study also found that hand washing rose by 34 per cent when a Jewish mother was either the patient or simply in the room as a visitor. No, the real stat is that hand washing rose by 34 per cent when the patient asked the health care worker to wash.

Become Dour and Dependable
A sixty-year-long study of a thousand people found that those who were conscientious as kids were 30 per cent less likely to die in any given year than were their more carefree peers. The same study also found that being cheerful in youth was correlated with a 6 per cent *increased* likelihood of dying in any given year. "Is that," you ask, "because the world really does suck?" Of course not. It's just that the terminally cheerful have a much higher rate of dying through strangulation by a close friend than do those who see the world the way it really is.

But what could account for dependable stay-at-home types living longer? A leading investigator concluded that it's probably because "squares" lead well-balanced, well-integrated lives. They are rarely diagnosed with a psychiatric ailment (and that's a good thing too because being a square is punishment enough, I think). They rarely abuse alcohol ("No, thank you. Tried it once, didn't like it."). They never use tranquillizers ("No, thank you. Tried it once, didn't like it."). And they also, of course, have only one child each.

Get a Pet
I have already told you that pets help lower stress levels in individuals, but they seem to do that for couples too. Karen Allen, a researcher from

the University of New York at Buffalo, did a study of one hundred couples, half of whom owned a cat or a dog. In data she presented to a meeting of the American Psychosomatic Society, she claims that the couples who owned pets are more happily married and respond better to stress.

Join a Church (Or Synagogue or Mosque or Temple or . . .)
There's lots of evidence about the benefits of this one. For example, a twenty-eight-year study from California concluded that people who attend church regularly live longer and healthier lives than those who are not religious about attending church. No one knows why this is so, but the authors speculate that the benefits of consistent religious participation, such as regular attendance at places of worship—churches, synagogues, mosques, temples, sports arenas—leads to an improved outlook, higher self-esteem, a sense of community, and encouragement from the other members of the religious institution to take better care of yourself. Another theory comes out of a study from Duke University that looked at elderly North Carolina residents and found that those who attended services at least once a week had better immune systems than non-churchgoing elderly North Carolinians. My own theory is much simpler, by the way. I think it's just that God wants to keep the true believers around longer.

But is that all the pro-prayer proof you can proffer, you agnostics may be wondering? As Marisa Tomei says in *My Cousin Vinny*, "No, there's more." In a review of over two hundred studies about religion, which was presented at a meeting of the American Association for the Advancement of Science, 75 per cent of the studies showed that religious commitment had positive effects on health and only 7 per cent showed that prayer was bad for your health, probably because those studies included lots of atheists and agnostics. The strongest positive effects on health, as one might expect, were on drug use, alcoholism, and depression, but religious commitment also seemed to have positive effects on diseases such as cancer, high blood pressure, and heart disease.

And for you cynics who want the benefits without the effort, I'm afraid that you have to be a committed believer to get those positive effects, because this study also concluded that those people who claim to pray at home actually have overall worse health outcomes than do the nonreligious.

One other thing you should know. If you can't pray or believe, it may not be your fault. It may all be in your genes. Some researchers are now claiming that they've found a "God spot" in the brain, a sort of religious G-spot, an area that seems to govern an innate belief in God, and it may just be that holy rollers are those people who have more cells in that particular area. The researchers claim that an area like that may have evolved because being religious adds stability to life and to society, although I figure it's just that God programmed it that way.

If You Won't Join a Church, Join Something Else, Anything
A report in the American Psychological Association's publication entitled *Psychological Bulletin* claims that belonging to something, anything, is a fundamental human need and that belonging to something improves both physical and mental health. Joining the drink-until-you-puke brotherhood at your local pub was probably not what these researchers had in mind, however.

If You Won't Join Something,
At Least Get a Friend to Go to Bingo with You
We need social support systems. Studies have shown, for example, that cancer patients in support groups can tolerate more chemotherapy than those not in support groups, that cancer patients in support groups generally have higher "natural killer cell" activity in their bodies, and that cancer patients in support groups have lower levels of cortisol, the main stress hormone. And if it's true for people with cancer, you can bet it's also true for people who are not as sick. Support and friends are vital to our well-being. Thus, elderly people who believe they are independent and who are surrounded by supportive, loving friends seem to live longer, while elderly men and women who have few social contacts, such as a spouse or friends, have twice the risk of dying as their same-age peers who maintain more social links with society. Bingo saves lives.

Now for the really fun bits, starting with advice on how to improve your love life.

Make More Money
Not only do the rich have more sex than those of us of lesser means (so just imagine what Bill Gates's love life must be like; better yet, don't),

but a 1996 American survey found that women worry more about money than do men, and women are more likely to think about money than sex—no surprise to most men, of course, although it may surprise some women that there are also some men who think about money more than sex. To underline how important money is, a study presented to a meeting of the American Psychological Association found that on the whole, for women, money is more important than a man's physical attraction, education, or occupation. That shouldn't really shock anyone, however, because if you have enough money, you can buy someone who has all the others.

Take Her Shopping More Often
A survey for the Factory Outlet Marketing Association found that 46 per cent of women would rather find a great bargain on clothes than have great sex.

Allow Her to Work in the Kitchen More Often
According to Dr. Jean Claude Kaufmann, a sociologist from the Sorbonne, housewives find that activities such as vacuuming and dusting provide "heightened emotions of love or hate" and that repeated participation in these activities leads to feelings that are akin to those experienced from erotic love. As a househusband of many years' standing, I have to say that this is probably one of those women things men can't relate to at all. I mean, when I'm home alone all day, I keep staring at that ironing board, but it never does anything for me.

Get Her Lots of Chocolate
You won't be surprised to learn, I'm sure, that a survey done, not coincidentally, for the Confectionery Manufacturers Association found that 38 per cent of Canadian women prefer chocolate to more sex, although you may be surprised to learn that 30 per cent of Canadian men made the same choice.

Get a Vasectomy
According to a survey done for Mary Stopes International, a British family planning charity, vasectomy is quick and painless and can improve your sex life. In fact, it's so pleasant that 92 per cent of men said they would recommend it to a friend. I agree. I recommend vasectomies

to all my friends, and one day I might even be brave enough to find out what one is really like.

Or a Personality

When *Psychology Today* readers were asked to rank the important features that would attract them to a man, women ranked intelligence first, sense of humour second, followed by ability to talk about feelings, ability to empathize, facial appearance, overall body build, sexual performance, and physical strength. The other feature mentioned by the authors as being more important than one might at first imagine was cleanliness (see "Wash Your Hands Constantly," above—and now I know why men should do it more often).

Become More Attractive

Besides cosmetic surgery and the subterfuge creams mentioned in Chapter 2, another form of camouflage is to buy garments that hide the true condition your condition is in. And lots of men seem to be doing that. A report in the *New York Times* claims that men are buying increasing numbers of such ego boosters as Slenderizing Manshape Undergarments, Super Shaper Briefs, and Butt Booster. What a joke, eh, and besides, my Manshapes were just so tight, they made my symptoms of gastrointestinal reflux disease much worse.

Rather than camouflage, some of you might prefer to concentrate on just becoming more symmetrical. It has been claimed, you see, that the most symmetrical faces are rated the most attractive: men with the most symmetrical faces lose their virginity earlier and tend to have more sexual partners than men whose nose is where their ear should be. And a study in the *New Scientist* claims that being symmetrical is better for your partner too. According to this study, if a woman's partner is "very symmetrical," women reach orgasm 75 per cent of the time, while with lopsided partners, they reach orgasm only 30 per cent of the time. That shouldn't be all that surprising, though. After all, common sense tells me that it's easier to reach orgasm when the person you're with looks more like someone from a Goya portrait than one straight out of a Picasso painting.

Smell Better

A study from Duke University looked at the effect that wearing cologne might have on a man's psychological health, and the researchers concluded that using pleasant odours does improve the mood of mid-life males." And if you're in a good mood and smelling good, hey, you're bound to be irresistible.

Another study, from the Smell and Taste Research Foundation in Chicago, claims that male sexual arousal can be turned on by fragrances such as the odours of pumpkin pie, donuts, licorice, and lavender, which can then send blood rushing to the penis. So who needs Viagra, eh? A couple of donuts and it's in the bag, guys.

Or You Could Just Smell Worse

A study from the Institute of Urban Ethology in Vienna found that women volunteers claimed that the more attractive a man's face was, the less appealing he smelled. So taking that to its logical conclusion, just try to smell awful, and women will find you irresistible, although I believe that this is a tactic already employed by many men, usually those in a slow-moving line in front of me.

Before you rush off to smell like a man's used locker, though, let me warn you that using smell to entice women is not as simple as it seems. You see, a study on cockroaches published in the journal *Nature* found that the difference between the male cockroaches on the top of the leftover pile in the kitchen and those on the bottom is usually a result of the scents the cockroaches give off. If a male gives off too much of a status-lowering scent, he quickly becomes a roach feeding off the crumbs left behind by the more dominant roaches. So why, you may wonder, has evolution allowed a status-lowering scent to persist? Because of female roaches, that's why. It turns out, you see, that some female roaches get turned on by the more vulnerable males. Sound familiar?

If nothing else works, you can always buy some Japanese underpants prelaced with sweat. Yes, the Japanese, patron saints of useless inventions, have invented underpants laced with artificial sweat containing a synthesized pheromone found in the sweat of the underarm. I've ordered eight pairs.

Best of All, Why Not Go Whole Hog?

Based on the responses obtained in sex surveys and findings from studies on sex (most of which have been cited earlier), here's what you do to increase your chances of having a lot of sex: buy as many jazz CD's as you can; get yourself a big gun or, even better, several; start smoking and drinking excessively; become a couch potato; buy yourself a trailer, but make sure to park it next to a Saks or Bloomingdale's store, where your mate can shop to her heart's content while you are busy buying her lots of household appliances; stock your trailer with tons of Swiss chocolate; rob a bank, but get shot while escaping so that you can seem more vulnerable; get as much plastic surgery as you can afford, including some more grey cells; get yourself fixed; learn to expose your female side; and smell worse.

What is sobering, though, is how many men already have many of those bases covered, and it still hasn't done them any good.

Have Lots and Lots of Orgasms
A study of middle-aged Welshmen from the town of Caerphilly and its environs found that the more orgasms a male has over a lifetime, the more likely he is to live longer. Now I realize that at first glance, this finding might run counter to my earlier speculations that chasing after too much sex might decrease one's life expectancy. But it doesn't, probably because several variables in this study had a strong bearing on these results. For example, men who reported more orgasms were also taller and healthier and had less risky jobs. More important, who ever said that frequency of orgasms had anything to do with sex? Especially for Welshmen.

Vote Conservative
British researchers from the University of Bristol have conducted a survey that shows that for nearly two decades, those Brits who voted Labour have a much greater chance of early death than do those who voted Tory. My theory is that it's because good Labourites refused to continue living under Margaret Thatcher's and John Major's oppressive regimes, or because they are now committing hara-kiri en masse after seeing what Tony Blair has done to their principles.

Start Revealing Everything
A survey from Santa Clara University that studied three hundred adults found that those who kept important secrets to themselves suffered more depression and anxiety, as well as aches and pains, than those who had spilled the beans. This finding also explains why women are so much healthier than men. In fact, if telling all your secrets is the real key to health, it's a wonder that women get sick at all.

If You Don't Have Something Nice to Say, Stow It

According to research presented in the *Journal of Personality and Social Psychology*, if you say something negative about someone, there is a strong tendency on the part of the listener to ascribe those traits to you. So if for some unfathomable reason you don't like this book, sit on it, OK? It's only going to boomerang on you if you say anything to someone. I tell you this only for your benefit.

Start Fooling Yourself

This one really works, and lots of people are doing it. A poll for Ortho Pharmaceuticals, for example, published in *USA Today* revealed that three in four baby boomers think they look younger than their age, and nearly 80 per cent of middle agers think their faces look younger than those of their peers.

But even if you can't stop looking your age, you can still fool yourself. Just push the goalposts farther out. And that's what most of us do, it seems, because according to that poll I just cited, the older boomers are, the later they say that middle age starts. Boomers who are thirty to thirty-four say that middle age starts at forty, while those who are already forty-five to fifty think that middle age really only starts at age forty-four. I think it starts at fifty-one-and-a-half.

Another good way to fool yourself and benefit from it is to tell yourself that no matter what your mother says, that girl you married is still a catch. A study in the *Journal of Personality and Social Psychology* concludes that people in the happiest relationships tend to see their partners through rose-coloured glasses, and that's what I keep telling my wife every time she wonders about me. "It's not me, dear. It's you. You're just wearing the wrong glasses today."

Do One Good Thing a Day

A study from the State University of New York at Stony Brook published in the journal *Health Psychology* shows that a small boost to the immune system that comes from doing something pleasant can last for up to two days. So go ahead. Start doing a few nice things a day. Put the toilet seat down once in a while, let the squeegee kid wash your windshield and give him a dime for his efforts. Believe me, you will feel so much better for being so nice. And the new friends you will make!

Lose Your Job

A study from the University of North Carolina suggests that contrary to what you might expect, losing one's job may contribute to a longer, healthier life for some people. Why? Well, I'm sure this is not going to surprise anyone who has ever spent any time in the company of young, happy, unemployed skiers, but this researcher concludes that most people are happier when they're not working. Not only that, work can be hazardous, work is often stressful, and work takes time, time that could be spent on exercise and making yourself healthy, which is exactly what I'm sure all those unemployed kids rush off to do as soon as they lose their jobs. So the more you work, the less healthy you may be. I had no trouble convincing my son about that one, of course.

Become a Shrinking Violet

British researchers claim that being submissive and having low self-confidence can reduce the risk of a heart attack, especially in women. That is why, as a husband very much interested in my wife's health, I pinned this finding to my fridge door. No luck, I'm afraid. My wife ripped it up and, well, I won't tell you the exact words she used, but suffice it to say that a shrinking violet would never have talked like that. Or sworn like that either.

Don't Go Anywhere Near a Certain Plastic Surgeon

Even if it is true that as a study found, well-hung guys are more likely to have more sex by being more promiscuous than guys with not as much to brag about, one thing I would advise you never to do is con-tact the Beverly Hills plastic surgeon who claims he can stretch your penis by attaching it to a bell-shaped weighted system, which, by the way, is available in two- and four-pound weights. Never mind about what you tell someone if one of those weights slips off and falls down your pants during an important business meeting. Of greater concern is what happens if it works too well. I mean, what if you stretch too much, and like an elastic, it refuses to retract again?

The Most Important Advice of All: Don't Feel So Guilty

A British study concluded that people the world over are plagued with guilt about smoking, eating, alcohol use, and exercise, and that guilt is producing lots of stress. So accept this absolution from me: Don't feel guilty. You did your best. Now enjoy your life.

Bibliography

This listing comprises the references that I consider most important, along with several review articles that might be of interest to readers.

CHAPTER 1

Allman, J., et al. 1998. Parenting and survival in anthropoid primates: Caretakers live longer. *Proc Natl Acad Sci USA* 95:6866–69.

Brim, O. 1996. Project explores landscape of midlife. *APA [American Psychological Association] Monitor*, November, 1.

Bumpass, L. 1994. *MIDMAC Bulletin* No. 2.

Burns-Cox, N., and C. Gingell. 1997. The andropause: Fact or fiction? *Postgrad Med* 73:553–56.

Cerha, J.R., and R.B. Wallace. 1997. Change in social ties and subsequent mortality in rural elders. *Epidemiology* 8:475–81.

Cockburn, J. and S. Pit. 1997. Prescribing behaviour in clinical practice: Patients' expectations and doctors' perceptions of patients' expectations—A questionnaire study. *BMJ* 315:520–25.

Diamond, J. 1997. *Male Menopause.* Naperville, Ill.: Sourcebooks Inc.

Director's notes. 1994–1996. *MIDMAC Bulletin*, Nos. 1–5.

Evans, R.G., et al. 1994. *Why Are Some People Healthy and Others Not? The Determinants of Health of Populations.* Hawthorne, N.Y.: Aldine de Gruyter.

Gallagher, W. 1993. Midlife myths. *The Atlantic Monthly,* May, 51–68.

Gonzales, R., et al. 1997. Antibiotic prescribing for adults with colds, upper respiratory tract infections, and bronchitis by ambulatory care physicians. *JAMA* 278:901–4.

Kruger, A. 1994. The midlife transition: Crisis or chimera. *Psychol Rep* 75:1299–1305.

Levenson, R.W., et al. 1993. Long-term marriage: Age, gender, satisfaction. *Psychol Aging* 8:301–13.

Lynch, J.W., et al. 1997. Cumulative impact of sustained economic hardship on physical, cognitive, psychological, and social functioning. *N Engl J Med* 337:1889–95.

Marmot, M.G. 1997. Contribution of job control and other risk factors to social variations in coronary heart disease incidence. *Lancet* 350:235–39.

Marmot, M.G. 1998. Improvement of social environment to improve health. *Lancet* 351:57–60.

Mookherjee, H.N. 1997. Marital status, gender, and perception of well-being. *J Soc Psychol* 137:95–105.

Mussen, P., et al. 1982. Early adult antecedents of life satisfaction at age 70. *J Gerontol* 37:316–22.

Orbuch, T.L., et al. 1996. Marital quality over the life course. *Social Psychology Quarterly* 59 (June):162.

Sheehy, G. 1998. *Understanding Men's Passages: Discovering the New Map of Men's Lives.* Toronto: Random House.

Shek, D.T. 1996. Midlife crisis in Chinese men and women. *J Psychol* 130:109–19.

Tucker, J.S., et al. 1996. Marital history at midlife as a predictor of longevity: Alternative explanations to the protective effect of marriage. *Health Psychol* 15:94–101.

Vaillant, C.O., and G.E. Vaillant. 1993. Is the U-curve of marital satisfaction an illusion? A 40-year study of marriage. *Journal of Marriage and the Family* 55:230–39.

CHAPTER 2

Coffey, C., et al. 1998. Sex differences in brain aging: A quantitative magnetic resonance imaging study. *Arch Neurol* 55:169–79.

Connor, S. 1996. Women win mental battle of sexes. *The Sunday Times,* 11 February, sec. 1, p. 7.

Cosmetic surgery with lasers. 1997. *Med Lett Drugs Ther* 39:10–12.

Cowell, P.E., et al. 1994. Sex differences in aging of the human frontal and temporal lobes. *J Neurosci* 14:4748–55.

Gur, R.C., et al. 1995. Sex differences in regional cerebral glucose metabolism during a resting state. *Science* 267:528–31.

Hawkes, N. 1997. Old people who stay healthy also stay sharp. *The Times,* 25 August, 6.

McClearn, G.E. 1997. Substantial genetic influence on cognitive abilities in twins 80 or more years old. *Science* 276:1560–63.

Medina, J. 1996. *The Clock of Ages: Why We Age, How We Age, Winding Back the Clock.* Cambridge: Cambridge University Press.

Meier, D.E., et al. 1987. Marked decline in trabecular bone mineral content in healthy men with age: Lack of association with sex steroid levels. *J Am Geriatr Soc* 35:189–97.

Morrison, J.H., and P.R. Hof. 1997. Life and death of neurons in the aging brain. *Science* 278:412–18.

Murphy, D.G., et al. 1996. Sex differences in human brain morphometry and metabolism: An in vivo quantitative magnetic resonance imaging and positron emission tomography study on the effect of aging. *Arch Gen Psychiatry* 53:585–94.

Orrell, M., et al. 1995. Education and dementia. *BMJ* 310:951–52.

Ott, A., et al. 1995. Prevalence of Alzheimer's disease and vascular dementia: Association with education. The Rotterdam study. *BMJ* 310:970–73.

Propecia and Rogaine Extra Strength for alopecia. 1998. *Med Lett Drugs Ther* 40:25–27.

Reed, R.L., et al. 1991. The relationship between muscle mass and muscle strength in the elderly. *J Am Geriatr Soc* 39:555–61.

Schiffman, S.S. 1997. Taste and smell losses in normal aging and disease. *JAMA* 278:1357–62.

Topical drugs for aging skin. 1997. *Med Lett Drugs Ther* 39:78–80.

Topical minoxidil for baldness: A reappraisal. 1994. *Med Lett Drugs Ther* 36:9–10.

CHAPTER 3

Hormones and Sexual Functioning

Adams, M.R., et al. 1995. Effects of androgens on coronary artery atherosclerosis and atherosclerosis-related impairment of vascular responsiveness. *Arterioscler Thromb Vasc Biol* 15:562–70.

Angier, N. 1995. Does testosterone equal aggression? Maybe not. *New York Times*, 20 June, A1, C3.

Bagatell, C.J., and W.J. Bremner. 1996. Androgens in men—Uses and abuses. *Drug Therapy* 334:707–14.

Bardin, C.W., et al. 1991. Androgens: Risks and benefits. *J Clin Endocrinol Metab* 73:4–7.

Behre, H.M., et al. 1994. Prostate volume in testosterone-treated and untreated hypogonadal men in comparison to age-matched controls. *Clin Endocrinol* (Oxford) 40:341–49.

Behre, H.M., et al. 1997. Long-term effect of testosterone therapy on bone mineral density in hypogonadal men. *J Clin Endocrinol Metab* 82:2386–90.

Bhasin, S., et al. 1997. Testosterone replacement increases fat-free mass and muscle size in hypogonadal men. *J Clin Endocrinol Metab* 82:407–13.

Booth, A., et al. 1989. Testosterone, and winning and losing in human competition. *Horm Behav* 23:556–71.

Breedlove, S.M. 1997. Sex on the brain. *Nature* 389:801.

Carruthers, M. 1996. *Male Menopause: Restoring Vitality and Virility.* New York: HarperCollins.

Dabbs, J.M., et al. 1997. Age, testosterone, and behaviour among female prison inmates. *Psychosom Med* 59:477–80.

Demark-Wahnefried, W., et al. 1997. Serum androgens: Association with prostate cancer risk and hair patterning. *J Androl* 18:495–500.

Halpern, C.T., et al. 1997. Testosterone predicts initiation of coitus in adolescent females. *Psychosom Med* 59:161–71.

Katznelson, L., et al. 1996. Increase in bone density and lean body mass during testosterone administration in men with acquired hypogonadism. *J Clin Endocrinol Metab* 81:4358–65.

Lakowski, B., and S. Hekimi. 1996. Determination of life-span in *Caenorhabditis elegans* by four clock genes. *Science* 272:1010–13.

Lamberts, S.W., et al. 1997. The endocrinology of aging. *Science* 278:419–24.

Masters, W., and V. Johnson. 1970. *Human Sexual Response.* Boston: Little, Brown.

Matsumato, A.M., et al. 1990. Effects of chronic testosterone administration in normal men: Safety and efficacy of high dosage testosterone and parallel dose-dependent suppression of luteinizing hormone, follicle-stimulating hormone, and sperm production. *J Clin Endocrinol Metab* 70:282–87.

Mazur, A., et al. 1980. Testosterone, status, and mood in human males. *Horm Behav* 14 (September):236–46.

Medina, J. 1996. *The Clock of Ages: Why We Age, How We Age, Winding Back the Clock.* Cambridge: Cambridge University Press.

Morley, J.E. 1991. Endocrine factors in geriatric sexuality. *Clin Geriatr Med* 7:85–93

Morley, J.E., et al. 1997. Longitudinal changes in testosterone, luteinizing hormone, and follicle-stimulating hormone in healthy older men. *Metabolism* 46:410–13.

Morley, J.E., et al. 1997. Potentially predictive and manipulable blood serum correlates of aging in the healthy human male: Progressive decreases in bioavailable testosterone, dehydroepiandrosterone sulfate, and the ratio of insulin-like growth factor 1 to growth hormone. *Proc Natl Acad Sci USA* 94:7537–42.

Motluk, A. 1997. Does lust for sex kill males in their prime? *New Scientist*, 24 May, 19.

Phillips, G.B., et al. 1994. The association of hypotestosteronemia with coronary artery disease in men. *Arterioscler Thromb* 14:701–6.

Quantum sufficit. 1995. *Am Fam Physician* 52:28.

Smith, T.W. 1992. Discrepancies between men and women in reporting number of sexual partners: A summary from four countries. *Soc Biol* 39 (Fall–Winter):203–11.

Tenover, J.L. 1992. Effects of testosterone supplementation in the aging male. *J Clin Endocrin Metab* 75:1092–98.

Tenover, J.L. 1997. Testosterone and the aging male. *J Androl* 18:103–6.

Testosterone patches for hypogonadism. 1996. *Med Lett Drugs Ther* 38:49–50.

Wang, C. 1995. Effect of testosterone replacement therapy on mood changes in hypogonadal men. Paper read at 77th Annual Meeting of the Endocrine Society, 14–17 June, Washington, D.C.

Wiederman, M.W. 1997. Extramarital sex: Prevalence and correlates in a national survey. *J Sex Res* 34:167–74.

Wiederman, M.W. 1997. The truth must be in there somewhere: Examining the gender discrepancy in self-reported lifetime number of sex partners. *J Sex Res* 34:375–86.

Zmuda, J.M., et al. 1996. Testosterone decreases lipoprotein(a) in men. *Am J Cardiol* 77:1244–47.

Zmuda, J.M., et al. 1997. Longitudinal relation between endogenous testosterone and cardiovascular disease risk factors in middle-aged men. A 13-year follow-up of former Multiple Risk Factor Intervention Trial participants. *Am J Epidemiol* 146:609–17.

Impotence

Dowd, M. 1998. Father's little helper. *New York Times* (late edn., East Coast), 26 April, sec. 4, p. 15.

Feldman, H.A., et al. 1994. Impotence and its medical and psychosocial correlates: Results of the Massachusetts Male Aging Study. *J Urol* 151:54–61.

Goldstein, I., et al. 1998. Oral sildenafil in the treatment of erectile dysfunction. Sildenafil Study Group. *N Engl J Med* 338:1397–404.

Gray, A., et al. 1991. Age, diseases and changing sex hormone levels in middle-aged men: Results of the Massachusetts Male Aging Study. *J Clin Endocrinol Metab* 73:1016–25.

Greco, E., and P. Poloni-Balbi. 1997. Penile rigidity in erectile dysfunction treated with alprostadil. *Lancet* 350:1682.

Intraurethral alprostadil for impotence. 1997. *Med Lett Drugs Ther* 39:32.

Kaiser, F.E., et al. 1988. Impotence and aging: Clinical and hormonal factors. *J Am Geriatr Soc* 36:511–19.

Korenman, S.G., et al. 1990. Secondary hypogonadism in older men: Its relation to impotence. *J Clin Endocrinol Metab* 71:963–69.

Morley, J.E., and F.E. Kaiser. 1993. Impotence: The internist's approach to diagnosis and treatment in advances. *Mosby Year Book*, edited by G.H. Stollerman, et al., 38:151–68.

Padma-Nathan, H., et al. 1997. Treatment of men with erectile dysfunction with transurethral alprostadil. Medicated Urethral System for Erection (MUSE) Study Group. *N Engl J Med* 336:1–7.

Sheehy, G. 1993. The unspeakable passage: Is there a male menopause? *Vanity Fair* (April):164–67, 218–27.

Sildenafil: An oral drug for impotence. 1998. *Med Lett Drugs Ther* 40:51–52.

Walker, C. 1997. Male stock hit by slump. *The Times*, 30 October, 17.

Yohimbine for male sexual dysfunction. 1994. *Med Lett Drugs Ther* 36:115–16.

CHAPTER 4

Benign Prostatic Hyperplasia

Barry, M.J., et al. 1997. The natural history of patients with benign prostatic hyperplasia as diagnosed by North American urologists. *J Urol* 157:10–15.

Benign Prostatic Hyperplasia Guideline Panel. 1994. Benign prostatic hyperplasia: Diagnosis and treatment. *Am Fam Physician* 49:1157–66.

Dahlstrund, C., et al. 1996. Snoring—a common cause of voiding disturbance in elderly men. *Lancet* 347:270–71.

Lepor, H., et al. 1996. The efficacy of terazosin, finasteride, or both in benign prostatic hyperplasia. Veterans Affairs Cooperative Studies Benign Prostatic Hyperplasia Study Group. *N Engl J Med* 335:533–39.

McAllister, J. 1996. TUNA may be new fish in prostate Rx pond. *Medical Post*, 2 July, 22.

McConnell, J.D., et al. 1998. The effect of finasteride on the risk of acute urinary retention and the need for surgical treatment among men with benign prostatic hyperplasia. Finasteride Long-Term Efficacy and Safety Study Group. *N Engl J Med* 338:557–63, 612–13.

The Prostatron: Microwaves for benign prostatic hyperplasia. 1996. *Med Lett Drugs Ther* 38:53–54.

Terazosin for benign prostatic hyperplasia. 1994. *Med Lett Drugs Ther* 36:15–16.

Wasson, J.H., et al. 1995. A comparison of transurethral surgery with watchful waiting for moderate symptoms of benign prostatic hyperplasia. Veterans Affairs Cooperative Study Group on Transurethral Resection of the Prostate. *N Engl J Med* 332:75–79, 99–109.

Prostate Cancer

Blasko, J.C., et al. 1997. Prostate cancer—the therapeutic challenge of locally advanced disease. *N Engl J Med* 337:340–41.

Carter, H.B., et al. 1997. Recommended prostate-specific antigen testing intervals for the detection of curable prostate cancer. *JAMA* 277:1456–60.

Catalona, W.J., et al. 1997. Prostate cancer detection in men with serum PSA concentrations of 2.6 to 4.0 ng/mL and benign prostate examination. *JAMA* 277:1452–55.

Chan, J.M., et al. 1998. Plasma insulin-like growth factor-I and prostate cancer risk: A prospective study. *Science* 279:563–66.

Collins, M.M., and M.J. Barry. 1996. Controversies in prostate cancer screening: Analogies to the early lung cancer screening debate. *JAMA* 276:1976–78.

Demark-Wahnefried, W., et al. 1997. Anthropometric risk factors for prostate cancer. *Nutr Cancer* 28:302–7.

Dietary factors play critical role in prostate cancer. 1996. *Medical Post*, 6 August, 28.

Frydenberg, M., et al. 1997. Prostate cancer diagnosis and management. *Lancet* 349:1681–87.

Gerber, G.S., et al. 1996. Results of radical prostatectomy in men with clinically localized prostate cancer. *JAMA* 276:615–19.

Goldenberg, S.L. 1992. *The Intelligent Patient Guide to Prostate Cancer: All You Need to Know to Take an Active Part in Your Treatment.* Vancouver: Intelligent Patient Guide.

Grönberg, H., et al. 1997. Characteristics of prostate cancer in families potentially linked to hereditary prostate cancer 1 (HPC 1) locus. *Jama* 278:1251–55.

Gunby, P. 1997. Prostate cancer's complexities of causation, detection, and treatment challenge researchers. *JAMA* 277:1580–82.

Heinonen, O.P., et al. 1998. Prostate cancer and supplementation with alpha-tocopherol and beta-carotene: Incidence and mortality in a controlled trial. *J Natl Cancer Inst* 90:414–15, 440–46.

Johansson, J.E., et al. 1997. Fifteen-year survival in prostate cancer. A prospective, population-based study in Sweden. *JAMA* 277:467–71, 97–98.

McLellan, D.L., and R.W. Norman. 1995. Hereditary aspects of prostate cancer. *Can Med Assoc J* 153:895–900.

Pace, K.T., and L.H. Klotz. 1997. PSA testing: Still controversial. *Canadian Journal of Diagnosis*, April, 67–75.

Screening cuts prostate cancer deaths: Study. 1998. *Medical Post*, 9 June, 32.

Stephenson, J. 1997. Health agencies update: Vitamin D and prostate cancer. *JAMA* 277:201.

Waxman, J., and D. Sheer. 1995. Is prostate cancer worth diagnosing? *Lancet* 346:1177–78.

Woodrum, D.L., et al. 1998. Interpretation of free prostate specific antigen clinical research studies for the detection of prostate cancer. *J Urol* 159 (January):5–12.

CHAPTER 5

McCormack, J., et al. 1996. *Drug Therapy Decision Making Guide.* Philadelphia: W.B. Saunders.

Rosenberg, M.W., and E.G. Moore. 1997. The health of Canada's elderly population: Current status and future implications. *Can Med Assoc J* 157:1025–32.

Alzheimer's

Connor, S. 1998. Vitamins could reduce risk of Alzheimer's disease. *The Sunday Times*, 26 April, sec. 1, p. 15.

Martyn A.D., et al. 1997. Aluminum concentrations in drinking water and risk of Alzheimer's disease. *Epidemiology* 8:281–86.

Ott, A., et al. 1995. Prevalence of Alzheimer's disease and vascular dementia: Association with education. The Rotterdam study. *BMJ* 310:970–73.

Petersen, R.C., et al. 1995. Apolipoprotein E status as a predictor of the development of Alzheimer's disease in memory-impaired individuals. *JAMA* 273:1274–78.

Sano, M., et al. 1997. A controlled trial of selegiline, alpha-tocopherol, or both as treatment for Alzheimer's disease. The Alzheimer's Disease Cooperative Study. *N Engl J Med* 336:1216–22, 1245–47.

Stewart, W.F., et al. 1997. Risk of Alzheimer's disease and duration of NSAID use. *Neurology* 48:626–32.

Whitehead, R., and C. Bates. 1997. Atherosclerosis, apolipoprotein E, and prevalence of dementia and Alzheimer's disease in the Rotterdam Study. *Lancet* 349:151–54.

Back Pain

Carey, T., et al. 1995. The outcomes and costs of care for acute low back pain among patients seen by primary care practitioners, chiropractors, and orthopedic surgeons. The North Carolina Back Pain Project. *N Engl J Med* 333:913–17.

Frost, H., et al. 1995. Randomised controlled trial for evaluation of fitness programme for patients with chronic low back pain. *BMJ* 310:151–54.

Jensen, M.C., et al. 1994. Magnetic resonance imaging of the lumbar spine in people without back pain. *N Engl J Med* 331:69–73, 115–16.

Malmivaara, A., et al. 1995. The treatment of acute low back pain—bed rest, exercises, or ordinary activity? *N Engl J Med* 332:351–55.

Depression

Barefoot, J., and M. Schroll. 1996. Symptoms of depression, acute myocardial infarction, and total mortality in a community sample. *Circulation* 93:1976–80.

Coulehan, J.L., et al. 1997. Treating depressed primary care patients improves their physical, mental, and social functioning. *Arch Intern Med* 157:1113–20.

Drugs for psychiatric disorders. 1997. *Med Lett Drugs Ther* 39:33–40.

Everson, S.A., et al. 1998. Depressive symptoms and increased risk of stroke mortality over a 29-year period. *Arch Intern Med* 158:1133–38.

Frasure-Smith, N., et al. 1993. Depression following myocardial infarction: Impact on 6-month survival. *JAMA* 270:1819–25.

Hirschfeld, R.M.A., et al. 1997. The National Depressive and Manic-Depressive Association consensus statement on the undertreatment of depression. *JAMA* 277:333–40.

Patrick-Cooper, L., et al. 1997. Exercise and depression in midlife: A prospective study. *Am J Public Health* 87:670–73.

Roose, S.P., et al. 1998. Comparison of paroxetine and nortriptyline in depressed patients with ischemic heart disease. *JAMA* 279:287–91.

Some drugs that cause psychiatric symptoms. 1998. *Med Lett Drugs Ther* 40:21–24.

St. John's wort. 1997. *Med Lett Drugs Ther* 39:107–9.

Wassertheil-Smoller, S., et al. 1996. Change in depression as a precursor of cardiovascular events. SHEP Cooperative Research Group (Systolic hypertension in the elderly). *Arch Intern Med* 156:553–61.

Weissman, M.M., et al. 1997. Offspring of depressed parents. 10 years later. *Arch Gen Psychiatry* 54:932–40.

Diabetes

The Diabetes Control and Complications Trial Research Group. 1993. The effect of intensive treatment of diabetes on the development and progression of long-term complications in insulin-dependent diabetes mellitus. *N Engl J Med* 329:977–86.

Ford, E.S., et al. 1997. Weight change and diabetes incidence: Findings from a national cohort of US adults. *Am J Epidemiol* 146:214–22.

Gaster, B., and I. Hirsch. 1998. The effects of improved glycemic control on complications in type 2 diabetes. *Arch Intern Med* 158:134–40.

Krolewski, A.S., et al. 1995. Glycosylated hemoglobin and the risk of microalbuminuria in patients with insulin-dependent diabetes mellitus. *N Engl J Med* 332:1251.

Leibson, C., et al. 1995. Adult-onset diabetes mellitus may increase risk of dementia. *Am Fam Physician* 52:1487.

Mayer-Davis, E.J., et al. 1998. Intensity and amount of physical activity in relation to insulin sensitivity: The Insulin Resistance Atherosclerosis Study. *JAMA* 279:669–74.

Gastroesophageal Reflux Disease

Harding, S., et al. 1996. Asthma and gastroesophageal reflux: Acid suppressive therapy improves asthma outcome. *Am J Med* 100:395–405.

Klinkenberg-Knol, E.C., et al. 1994. Long-term treatment with omeprazole for refractory reflux esophagitis: Efficacy and safety. *Ann Intern Med* 121:161–67.

Over-the-counter H2-receptor antagonists for heartburn. 1995. *Med Lett Drugs Ther* 37:95–96.

Heart Disease

Allen, J.K., et al. 1996. Prevalence of hypercholesterolemia among siblings of persons with premature coronary heart disease. Application of the Second Adult Treatment Panel guidelines. *Arch Intern Med* 156:1654–60.

Barker, D.J. 1995. Fetal origins of coronary heart disease. *BMJ* 311:171–74.

Benfante, R., et al. 1994. To what extent do cardiovascular risk factor values measured in elderly men represent their midlife values measured 25 years earlier? A preliminary report and commentary from the Honolulu Heart Program. *Am J Epidemiol* 140:206–16.

Breteler, M.B., et al. 1994. Cardiovascular disease and distribution of cognitive function in elderly people: The Rotterdam Study. *BMJ* 308:1604–8.

Byington, R., et al. 1995. Reduction in cardiovascular events during pravastatin therapy. Pooled analysis of clinical events of the Pravastatin Atherosclerosis Intervention Program. *Circulation* 92:2419–25.

Choice of lipid-lowering drugs. 1996. *Med Lett Drugs Ther* 38:67–70.

De Lorgeril, M., et al. 1998. Mediterranean dietary pattern in a randomized trial: Prolonged survival and possible reduced cancer rate. *Arch Intern Med* 158:1181–87.

Downs, J.R., et al. 1998. Primary prevention of acute coronary events with lovastatin in men and women with average cholesterol levels: Results of AFCAPS/ TexCAPS. Air Force/Texas Coronary Atherosclerosis Prevention Study. *JAMA* 279:1615–22, 59–61.

Gaziano, J.M., et al. 1997. Fasting triglycerides, high-density lipoprotein, and risk of myocardial infarction. *Circulation* 96:2520–25.

Gillman, M.W., et al. 1997. Margarine intake and subsequent coronary heart disease in men. *Epidemiology* 8:144–49.

Golomb, B.A. 1998. Cholesterol and violence: Is there a connection? *Ann Intern Med* 128:478–87.

Gotto, A.M., Jr. 1998. Triglyceride: The forgotten risk factor. *Circulation* 97:1027–36.

Graham, I.M., et al. 1997. Plasma homocysteine as a risk factor for vascular disease. The European Concerted Action Project. *JAMA* 277:1775–81.

Grover, S.A., et al. 1994. Serum lipid screening to identify high-risk individuals for coronary death. The results of the Lipid Research Clinics prevalence cohort. *Arch Intern Med* 154:679–84.

Hawkes, N. 1998. Slim chance of happiness on a low-fat diet. *The Times*, 30 January, 5.

Hennekens, C.H. 1998. Increasing burden of cardiovascular disease: Current knowledge and future directions for research on risk factors. *Circulation* 97:1095–1102.

Homocysteine Lowering Trialists Collaboration. 1998. Lowering blood homocysteine with folic acid based supplements: Meta-analysis of randomised trials. *BMJ* 316:894–98.

Jousilahti, P., et al. 1998. Serum cholesterol distribution and coronary heart disease risk: Observations and predictions among middle-aged population in eastern Finland. *Circulation* 97:1087–94.

Klag, M.J., et al. 1993. Serum cholesterol in young men and subsequent cardio-vascular disease. *N Engl J Med* 328:313–18.

Law, M.R., et al. 1994. Assessing possible hazards of reducing serum cholesterol. *BMJ* 308:373–79.

McCarron, D.A., et al. 1997. Nutritional management of cardiovascular risk factors. A randomized clinical trial. *Arch Intern Med* 157:169–77.

Miwa, K., et al. 1996. Vitamin E deficiency in variant angina. *Circulation* 94:14–18.

Muller, J.E., et al. 1996. Triggering myocardial infarction by sexual activity. Low absolute risk and prevention by regular physical exertion. Determinants of Myocardial Infarction Onset Study Investigators. *JAMA* 275:1405–9.

The Multiple Risk Factor Intervention Trial Research Group. 1996. Mortality after 16 years for participants randomized to the Multiple Risk Factor Intervention Trial. *Circulation* 94:946–51.

Omenn, G.S., et al. 1998. Preventing coronary heart disease: B vitamins and homocysteine. *Circulation* 97:421–24.

Siscovick, D.S., et al. 1995. Dietary intake and cell membrane levels of long-chain n-3 polyunsaturated fatty acids and the risk of primary cardiac arrest. *JAMA* 274:1363–67.

Tuomainen, T.P., et al. 1998. Association between body iron stores and the risk of acute myocardial infarction in men. *Circulation* 97:1461–66.

Verschuren, W.M.M., et al. 1995. Serum total cholesterol and long-term coronary heart disease mortality in different cultures: Twenty-five-year follow-up of the Seven Countries Study. *JAMA* 274:131–36.

Wardle, J., et al. 1996. Randomised placebo controlled trial of effect on mood of lowering cholesterol concentration. Oxford Cholesterol Study Group. *BMJ* 313:75–78.

Willerson, J.T. 1996. Effect of pravastatin on coronary events after myocardial infarction in patients with average cholesterol levels. *Circulation* 94:3054.

High Blood Pressure

Appel, L.J., et al. 1997. A clinical trial of the effects of dietary patterns on blood pressure. DASH Collaborative Research Group. *N Engl J Med* 336:1117–24.

Bulpitt, C.J., et al. 1994. Optimal blood pressure control in treated hypertensive patients. Report from the Department of Health Hypertension Care Computing Project (DHCCP). *Circulation* 90:225–33.

Drugs for hypertension. 1995. *Med Lett Drugs Ther* 37:45–50.

Elliot, P., et al. 1996. Intersalt revisited: Further analyses of 24 hour sodium excretion and blood pressure within and across populations. Intersalt Cooperative Research Group. *BMJ* 312:1249–53.

Kilander, L., et al. 1998. Hypertension is related to cognitive impairment: A 20-year follow-up of 999 men. *Hypertension* 31:780–86.

Launer, L.J., et al. 1995. The association between midlife blood pressure levels and late-life cognitive function. The Honolulu-Asia Aging Study. *JAMA* 274:1846–51.

Le Pailleur, C., et al. 1998. The effects of talking, reading, and silence on the "white coat" phenomenon in hypertensive patients. *Am J Hypertens* 11:203–7.

O'Donnell, C.J., et al. 1997. Hypertension and borderline isolated systolic hypertension increase risks of cardiovascular disease and mortality in male physicians. *Circulation* 95:1132–37.

Palatini, P., et al. 1998. Target-organ damage in stage I hypertensive subjects with white coat and sustained hypertension: Results from the HARVEST study. *Hypertension* 31:57–63.

Prospective Studies Collaboration. 1995. Cholesterol, diastolic blood pressure, and stroke: 13,000 strokes in 450,000 people in 45 prospective cohorts. *Lancet* 346:1647–53.

Safety of calcium-channel blockers. 1997. *Med Lett Drugs Ther* 39:13–14.

Sung, B.H., et al. 1997. Effects of cholesterol reduction on BP response to mental stress in patients with high cholesterol. *Am J Hypertens* 10:592–99.

Sytkowski, P., et al. 1996. Secular trends in long-term sustained hypertension, long-term treatment, and cardiovascular mortality. The Framingham Heart Study 1950 to 1990. *Circulation* 93:697–703.

Whelton, P.K., et al. 1997. Effects of oral potassium on blood pressure. Meta-analysis of randomized controlled clinical trials. *JAMA* 277:1624–32.

Stress

Leake, J., and C. Norton. 1998. Bad drivers are crashing bores in bed. *The Sunday Times*, 3 May, sec. 1, p. 13.

Blumenthal, J.A., et al. 1997. Stress management and exercise training in cardiac patients with myocardial ischemia. Effects on prognosis and evaluation of mechanisms. *Arch Intern Med* 157:2213–23.

Carney, R. 1998. Psychological risk factors for cardiac events: Could there be just one? *Circulation* 37:128–29.

Denollet, J., et al. 1996. Personality as independent predictor of long-term mortality in patients with coronary heart disease. *Lancet* 347:417–21.

Everson, A., et al. 1997. Hostility and increased risk of mortality and acute myocardial infarction: The mediating role of behavioral risk factors. *Am J Epidemiol* 146:142–52.

Friedman, H.S., and S. Booth-Kewley. 1988. Validity of the type A construct: A reprise. *Psychol Bull* 104:381–84.

Gabbay, F.H., et al. 1996. Triggers of myocardial ischemia during daily life in patients with coronary artery disease: Physical and mental activities, anger and smoking. *J Am Coll Cardiol* 27:585–92.

Gullette, E.C.D., et al. 1997. Effects of mental stress on myocardial ischemia during daily life. *JAMA* 277:1521–26.

Gump, B.B., and K.A. Matthews. 1998. Vigilance and cardiovascular reactivity to subsequent stressors in men: A preliminary study. *Health Psychol* 17:93–96.

Houston, B.K., et al. 1997. Social dominance and 22-year all-cause mortality in men. *Psychosom Med* 59:51–57.

Jiang, W.J., et al. 1996. Mental stress-induced myocardial ischemia and cardiac events. *JAMA* 275:1651–56.

Kamarck, T., et al. 1997. Exaggerated blood pressure responses during mental stress are associated with enhanced carotid atherosclerosis in middle-aged Finnish men: Findings from the Kuopio Ischemic Heart Disease Study. *Circulation* 96:3842–48.

Kubzansky, L., et al. 1997. Is worrying bad for your heart? A prospective study of worry and coronary heart disease in the Normative Aging Study. *Circulation* 95:818–24.

Markovitz, J.H., et al. 1993. Psychological predictors of hypertension in the Framingham Study. Is there tension in hypertension? *JAMA* 270:2439–43.

Marmot, M.G., et al. 1997. Contribution of job control and other risk factors to social variations in coronary heart disease incidence. *Lancet* 350:235–39.

Mittleman, M.A., et al. 1997. Educational attainment, anger, and the risk of triggering myocardial infarction onset. The Determinants of Myocardial Infarction Onset Study Investigators. *Arch Intern Med* 157:769–75.

Muller, J.A. 1996. Triggering myocardial infarction by sexual activity. Low absolute risk and prevention by regular physical exertion. Determinants of Myocardial Infarction Onset Study Investigators. *JAMA* 275:1405–9.

Murray, I. 1998. Health risk to staff who say: Have a nice day. *The Times*, 7 January, 6.

Suarez, E.C., et al. 1997. The relationship between hostility and beta-adrenergic receptor physiology in healthy young males. *Psychosom Med* 59:481–87.

Suarez, E.C., et al. 1998. Neuroendocrine, cardiovascular, and emotional responses of hostile men: The role of interpersonal challenge. *Psychosom Med* 60:78–88.

Theorell, T., et al. 1998. Decision latitude, job strain, and myocardial infarction: A study of working men in Stockholm. Stockholm Heart Epidemiology Program. *Am J Public Health* 88:382–88.

Osteoarthritis

Drugs for rheumatoid arthritis. 1994. *Med Lett Drugs Ther* 36:101–2.

Glucosamine for osteoarthritis. 1997. *Med Lett Drugs Ther* 39:91–92.

Jamison, R.N. 1995. Weather changes and pain: Perceived influence of local climate on pain complaint in chronic pain patients. *Pain* 61:309–15.

McAlindon, T., and D.T. Felson. 1997. Nutrition: Risk factors for osteoarthritis. *Ann Rheum Dis* 56:397–402.

Meyer, H.E., et al. 1996. Body height, body mass index, and fatal hip fractures:

16 years' follow-up of 674,000 Norwegian women and men. *Epidemiology* 6:299–305.

Osteoporosis

Burger, H., et al. 1998. Risk factors for increased bone loss in an elderly population: The Rotterdam Study. *Am J Epidemiol* 147:871–79.

Naves, M. 1997. The influence of alcohol consumption on the risk of vertebral deformity. European Vertebral Osteoporosis Study Group. *Osteoporos Int* 7(1):65–71.

Ooms, M., et al. 1995. Prevention of bone loss by vitamin D supplementation in elderly women: A randomized double-blind trial. *J Clin Endocrinol Metab* 80:1052–58.

Stroke

Pancioli, A.M., et al. 1998. Public perception of stroke warning signs and knowledge of potential risk factors. *JAMA* 279:1288–92.

CHAPTER 6

Buske, L. 1997. Canada's changing life-expectancy trends. *Can Med Assoc J* 157:1324.

Finch, C.E., and R.E. Tanzi. 1997. Genetics of aging. *Science* 278:407–23.

Khaw, K.T. 1997. Healthy aging. *BMJ* 315:1090–96.

Manton, K.G. 1997. Chronic disability trends in elderly United States populations: 1982–1994. *Proc Natl Acad Sci USA* 94:2593–98.

Rowe, J.W., and R.L. Kahn. 1998. *Successful Aging.* New York: Pantheon Books.

Successful aging. 1997. *Science* 278:407–23.

Vita, A.J., et al. 1998. Aging, health risks, and cumulative disability. *N Engl J Med* 338:1035–41.

Alcohol

Dent, O.F., et al. 1997. Alcohol consumption and cognitive performance in a random sample of Australian soldiers who served in the Second World War. *BMJ* 314:1655–57.

Doll, R., et al. 1994. Mortality in relation to consumption of alcohol: 13 years' observations on male British doctors. *BMJ* 309:911–18.

Dufouil, C., et al. 1997. Sex differences in the association between alcohol consumption and cognitive performance. *Am J Epidemiol* 146:405–12.

Duncan, B.B., et al. 1995. Association of the waist-to-hip ratio is different with wine than with beer or hard liquor consumption. Atherosclerosis Risk in Communities Study Investigators. *Am J Epidemiol* 142:1034–38.

Fillmore, K.M., et al. 1998. Alcohol consumption and mortality. I. Characteristics of drinking groups. *Addiction* 93:183–203.

Gaziano, J.M., et al. 1993. Moderate alcohol intake, increased levels of high-density lipoprotein and its subfractions, and decreased risk of myocardial infarction. *N Engl J Med* 329:1829–34.

Holbrook, T., and E. Barrett-Connor. 1993. A prospective study of alcohol consumption and bone mineral density. *BMJ* 306:1506–9.

Jensen, G.B., et al. 1993. Do alcoholics drink their neurons away? *Lancet* 342:1201–4.

Kauhanen, J. 1997. Beer binging and mortality: Results from the Kuopio ischaemic heart disease risk factor study, a prospective population based study. *BMJ* 315:846–51.

Kauhanen, J., et al. 1997. Frequent hangovers and cardiovascular mortality in middle-aged men. *Epidemiology* 8:281–86.

Klatsky, A.L., et al. 1997. Red wine, white wine, liquor, beer, and risk for coronary artery disease hospitalization. *Am J Cardiol* 80:416–20.

Lam, T.H. 1997. Relative risks are inflated in published literature. *BMJ* 315:880.

Marmot, M.G., et al. 1994. Alcohol and blood pressure: The INTERSALT study. *BMJ* 308:1263–67.

McElduff, P., and A.J. Dobson. 1997. How much alcohol and how often? Population based case-control study of alcohol consumption and risk of a major coronary event. *BMJ* 314:1159–64.

Rehm, J., et al. 1997. Alcohol consumption and coronary heart disease morbidity and mortality. *Am J Epidemiol* 146:495–501.

Renaud S.C., et al. 1998. Alcohol and mentality in middle-aged men from eastern France. *Epidemiology* 9:184–88.

Rimm, E.B., et al. 1996. Review of moderate alcohol consumption and reduced risk of coronary heart disease: Is the effect due to beer, wine, or spirits? *BMJ* 312:731–41.

Rivara, F.P., et al. 1997. Alcohol and illicit drug abuse and the risk of violent death in the home. *JAMA* 278:569–75.

Thun, M.J., et al. 1997. Alcohol consumption and mortality among middle-aged and elderly U.S. adults. *N Engl J Med* 337:1705–14.

Update: Alcohol-related traffic crashes and fatalities among youth and young adults—United States 1982–94. 1995. *MMWR Morb Mortal Wkly Rep* 44:869–74.

ASA

Aspirin for prevention of myocardial infarction. 1995. *Med Lett Drugs Ther* 37:14–16.

Brink, S. 1995. Pop an aspirin if the earth moves? *U.S. News and World Report*, 10 July, 53.

Col, N.F., et al. 1995. Does aspirin consumption affect the presentation or severity of acute myocardial infarction? *Arch Intern Med* 155:1386–89.

Lee, M., et al. 1994. Dose effects of aspirin on gastric prostaglandins and stomach mucosal injury. *Ann Intern Med* 120:184–89.

Savon, J.J., et al. 1995. Gastrointestinal blood loss with low dose (325 mg) plain and enteric-coated aspirin administration. *Am J Gastroenterol* 90:581–85.

Steering Committee of the Physicians' Health Study Research Group. 1989. Final report on the aspirin component of the ongoing Physicians' Health Study. *N Engl J Med* 321:129–35.

Valles, J., et al. 1998. Erythrocyte promotion of platelet reactivity decreases the effectiveness of aspirin as an antithrombotic therapeutic modality: The effect of low-dose aspirin is less than optimal in patients with vascular disease due to pro-thrombotic effects of erythrocytes on platelet reactivity. *Circulation* 97:350–55.

Weil, J., et al. 1995. Prophylactic aspirin and risk of peptic ulcer bleeding. *BMJ* 310:827–30.

Coffee

Kawachi, I., et al. 1996. A prospective study of coffee drinking and suicide in women. *Arch Intern Med* 156:521–25.

Brody, J.E. 1995. The latest news on coffee? Don't worry. Drink up. 1995. *New York Times* (late edn.), 13 September, C1, C6.

Sung, B.H. 1995. Caffeine elevates blood pressure response to exercise in mild hypertensive men. *Am J Hypertens* 8:1184–88.

Willett, W.C., et al. 1996. Coffee consumption and coronary heart disease in women. A ten-year follow-up. *JAMA* 275:458–62.

Diet

Albert, C.M., et al. 1998. Fish consumption and risk of sudden cardiac death. *JAMA* 279:23–28.

Council on Scientific Affairs. 1989. Dietary fiber and health. *JAMA* 262:542–46.

De Lorgeril, M., et al. 1996. Effect of a Mediterranean type of diet on the rate of cardiovascular complications in patients with coronary artery disease. *J Am Coll Cardiol* 28:1103–8.

Franceschi, S., et al. 1998. Role of different types pf vegetables and fruit in the prevention of cancer of the colon, rectum, and breast. *Epidemiology* 9:338–41.

Gillman, M.W., et al. 1995. Protective effect of fruits and vegetables on development of stroke in men. *JAMA* 273:1113–17.

Gillman, M.W., et al. 1997. Inverse association of dietary fat with development of ischemic stroke in men. *JAMA* 278:2145–50.

Hawkes, N. 1998. Slim chance of happiness on a low-fat diet. *The Times*, 30 January, 5.

Huijbregts, P., et al. 1997. Dietary pattern and 20 year mortality in elderly men in Finland, Italy, and the Netherlands: Longitudinal cohort study. *BMJ* 315:13–17.

Knopp, R.H., et al. 1997. Long-term cholesterol-lowering effects of 4 fat-restricted diets in hypercholesterolemic and combined hyperlipidemic men. The Dietary Alternatives Study. *JAMA* 278:1509–15.

Kohlmeier, L., et al. 1997. Lycopene and myocardial infarction risk in the EURAMIC Study. *Am J Epidemiol* 146:618–26.

Lane, M. 1996. Calorie restriction lowers body temperature in rhesus monkeys, consistent with a postulated anti-aging mechanism in rodents. *Proc Natl Acad Sci USA* 93:4159–64.

Le Marchon, L., et al. 1997. Dietary fiber and colorectal cancer risk. *Epidemiology* 8:658–65.

Pietinen, D., et al. 1996. Intake of dietary fiber and risk of coronary heart disease in a cohort of Finnish men. The Alpha-Tocopherol, Beta-Carotene Cancer Prevention Study. *Circulation* 94:2720–27, 2696–98.

Ruxton, C.H.S., and T.R. Kirk. 1997. Breakfast: A review of associations with measures of dietary intake, physiology and biochemistry. *Br J Nutr* 78:199–213.

Thorogood, M., et al. 1994. Risk of death from cancer and ischaemic heart disease in meat and non-meat eaters. *BMJ* 308:1667–70.

Weindruch, R., et al. 1997. Seminars in medicine of the Beth Israel Deaconess Medical Center. Caloric intake and aging. *New Engl J Med* 337:986–94.

Zino, S., et al. 1997. Randomised controlled trial of effect of fruit and vegetable consumption on plasma concentrations of lipids and antioxidants. *BMJ* 314:1787–91.

Supplements

The Alpha-Tocopherol, Beta Carotene Cancer Prevention Study Group. 1994. The effect of vitamin E and beta carotene on the incidence of lung cancer and other cancers in male smokers. *N Engl J Med* 330:1029–35.

Clark, L.C., et al. 1996. Effects of selenium supplementation for cancer prevention in patients with carcinoma of the skin. A randomized controlled trial. Nutritional Prevention of Cancer Study Group. *JAMA* 276:1957–63.

Connor, S. 1998. Vitamins could reduce risk of Alzheimer's disease. *The Sunday Times*, 26 April, sec. 1, p. 15.

Daviglus, M.L., et al. 1996. Beta-carotene, vitamin C and risk of prostate cancer: Results from the Western Electorc Study. *Epidemiology* 5:472–77.

Dehydroepiandrosterone (DHEA). 1996. *Med Lett Drugs Ther* 38:91–92.

Devaraj, S., et al. 1997. Dose-response comparison of RRR-alpha-tocopherol and all-racemic alpha-tocopherol on LDL oxidation. *Arterioscler Thromb Vasc Biol* 17:2273–79.

Khaw, K.T., and P. Woodhouse. 1995. Interrelation of vitamin C, infection, haemostatic factors, and cardiovascular disease. *BMJ* 310:1548–49, 1559–66.

Le Bars, P.L., et al. 1997. A placebo-controlled, double-blind, randomized trial of an extract of Ginkgo biloba for dementia. North American EGb Study Group. *JAMA* 278:1327–32.

Mark, S.D., et al. 1998. Do nutritional supplements lower the risk of stroke or hypertension? *Epidemiology* 9:9–15.

Nyyssonen, K., et al. 1997. Vitamin C deficiency and risk of myocardial infarction: Prospective population study of men from eastern Finland. *BMJ* 314:634–38.

Riemersma, R.A. 1996. Coronary heart disease and vitamin E. *Lancet* 347:776–77.

Sahyoun, N.R., et al. 1996. Carotenoids, vitamins C and E, and mortality in an elderly population. *Am J Epidemiol* 144:501–11.

Vita, J.A., et al. 1998. Low plasma ascorbic acid independently predicts the presence of an unstable coronary syndrome. *J Am Coll Cardiol* 31:980–86.

Watson, K., et al. 1997. Active serum vitamin D levels are inversely correlated with coronary calcification. *Circulation* 96:1755–60.

Whitehead, R., and C. Bates. 1997. Recommendations on folate intake. *Lancet* 350:1642.

CHAPTER 7

Fitness

Blair, S.N., et al. 1996. Influences of cardiorespiratory fitness and other precursors on cardiovascular disease and all-cause mortality in men and women. *JAMA* 276:205–10.

Fries, J.F., et al. 1994. Running and the development of disability with age. *Ann Intern Med* 121:502–9.

Hakim, A.A., et al. 1998. Effects of walking on mortality among nonsmoking retired men. *N Engl J Med* 338:94–99.

Hambrecht, R., et al. 1993. Various intensities of leisure time physical activity in patients with coronary artery disease: Effects on cardiorespiratory fitness and progression of coronary atherosclerotic lesions. *J Am Coll Cardiol* 22:468–77.

King, A.C., et al. 1997. Moderate-intensity exercise and self-rated quality of sleep in older adults. A randomized controlled trial. *JAMA* 277:32–37.

Kujala, V.M., et al. 1998. Relationship of leisure-time physical activity and mortality: The Finnish twin cohort. *JAMA* 279:440–44.

Lee, I.M., et al. 1995. Exercise intensity and longevity in men: The Harvard Alumni Health Study. *JAMA* 273:1179–84.

Mittleman, M.A., et al. 1993. Triggering of acute myocardial infarction by heavy physical exertion. Protection against triggering by regular exertion. Determinants of Myocardial Infarction Onset Study Investigators. *N Engl J Med* 329:1677–83.

Neeper, S.A., et al. 1995. Exercise and brain neurotrophins. *Nature* 373:109.

Quantum sufficit. 1996. *Am Fam Physician* 53:1494.

Wannamathee, S.G., et al. 1998. Changes in physical activity, mortality, and incidence of coronary heart disease in older men. *Lancet* 351:1603–8.

Williams, P.T. 1997. Relationship of distance run per week to coronary heart disease risk factors in 8283 male runners. The National Runners' Health Study. *Arch Intern Med* 157:191–98.

Williams, P.T. 1998. Relationships of heart disease risk factors to exercise quantity and intensity. *Arch Intern Med* 158:237–45.

Sleep

Braver, H.M., et al. 1995. Treatment for snoring. Combined weight loss, sleeping on side, and nasal spray. *Chest* 107:1283–88.

Breslau, N., et al. 1997. Daytime sleepiness: An epidemiological study of young adults. *Am J Public Health* 10:1649–53.

Bursztyn, M., et al. 1994. Siesta and ambulatory blood pressure monitoring. Comparability of the afternoon nap and night sleep. *Am J Hypertens* 7:217–21.

Chang, P.P., et al. 1997. Insomnia in young men and subsequent depression. The Johns Hopkins Precursors Study. *Am J Epidemiol* 146:105–14.

Coren, S. 1996. *Sleep Thieves: An Eye-Opening Exploration into the Science and Mysteries of Sleep*. New York: The Free Press.

Dawson, D., and K. Reid. 1997. Fatigue, alcohol and performance impairment. *Nature* 388:235.

Hypnotic drugs. 1996. *Med Lett Drugs Ther* 38:59–61.

Karni, A., et al. 1994. Dependence on REM sleep of overnight improvement of a perceptual skill. *Science* 265:679–82.

King, A.C., et al. 1997. Moderate-intensity exercise and self-rated quality of sleep in older adults. A randomized controlled trial. *JAMA* 277:32–37.

Kuppermann, M., et al. 1995. Sleep problems and their correlates in a working population. *J Gen Intern Med* 10:25–32.

Melatonin. 1995. *Med Lett Drugs Ther* 37:111–12.

Monk, T.H., et al. 1997. The effects on human sleep and circadian rhythms of 17 days of continuous bedrest in the absence of daylight. *Sleep* 20:858–64.

Netzer N., et al. 1998. Blood flow of the middle cerebral artery with sleep-disordered breathing: Correlation with obstructive hypopneas. *Stroke* 29:87–93.

Ohayon, M.M., et al. 1997. How sleep and mental disorders are related to complaints of daytime sleepiness. *Arch Intern Med* 157:2645–52.

Pressman, M.R., et al. 1996. Nocturia: A rarely recognized symptom of sleep apnea and other occult sleep disorders. *Arch Intern Med* 156:545–50.

Reilly, T., et al. 1997. Aging, rhythms of physical performance, and adjustment to changes in the sleep-activity cycle. *Occup Environ Med* 54:812–16.

Sharpley, A. 1996. Impact of daytime sleepiness underrated. *Lancet* 348:71.

Wilson, M.A., and B.L. McNaughton. 1994. Reactivation of hippocampal ensemble memories during sleep. *Science* 655:676–79.

Wright, J., et al. 1997. Health effects of obstructive sleep apnoea and the effectiveness of continuous positive airways pressure: A systematic review of the research evidence. *BMJ* 314:851–60.

Young, T., et al. 1997. Population-based study of sleep-disordered breathing as a risk factor for hypertension. *Arch Intern Med* 157:1746–52.

Smoking

Doll, R., et al. 1994. Mortality in relation to smoking: 40 years' observations on male British doctors. *BMJ* 309:901–11.

Fontham, E.Y.H., et al. 1994. Environmental tobacco smoke and lung cancer in nonsmoking women. A multicenter study. *JAMA* 271:1752–59.

Howard, G., et al. 1998. Cigarette smoking and progression of atherosclerosis: The Atherosclerosis Risk in Communities (ARIC) Study. *JAMA* 279:119–24.

Law, M., and J.L. Tang. 1995. An analysis of the effectiveness of interventions intended to help people stop smoking. *Arch Intern Med* 155:1933–41.

Stress

Berkman, L.F. 1998. Psychosocial experiences influence functioning: New risks, new outcomes. *Psychosom Med* 60:256–57.

Christenfeld, N., et al. 1997. Social support effects on cardiovascular reactivity: Is a stranger as effective as a friend? *Psychosom Med* 59:388–98.

Everson, S.A., et al. 1996. Hopelessness and risk of mortality and incidence of myocardial infarction and cancer. *Psychosom Med* 58:113–21.

Everson, S.A., et al. 1997. Interaction of workplace demands and cardiovascular reactivity in progression of carotid atherosclerosis: Population based study. *BMJ* 314:553–58.

Kiecolt-Glaser, J.K., et al. 1997. Marital conflict in older adults: Endocrinological and immunological correlates. *Psychosom Med* 59:339–49.

Lupien, S.J., et al. 1997. Stress-induced declarative memory impairment in healthy elderly subjects: Relationship to cortisol reactivity. *J Clin Endocrinol Metab* 82:2070–75.

Lynch, J.W., et al. 1997. Cumulative impact of sustained economic hardship on physical, cognitive, psychological, and social functioning. *N Engl J Med* 337:1889–95.

McEwen, B.S. 1998. Protective and damaging effects of stress mediators. *N Engl J Med* 338:171–79.

Penninx, B.W., et al. 1997. Effects of social support and personal coping resources on mortality in older age: The Longitudinal Aging Study Amsterdam. *Am J Epidemiol* 146:510–19.

Robinson-Whelen, S., et al. 1997. Distinguishing optimism from pessimism in older adults: Is it more important to be optimistic or not to be pessimistic? *J Pers Soc Psychol* 73:1345–53.

Russek, L.G., and G.E. Schwartz. 1997. Feelings of parental caring predict health status in midlife: A 35-year follow-up of the Harvard Mastery of Stress Study. *J Behav Med* 20:1–13.

Self-reported frequent mental distress among adults—United States, 1993–1996. 1998. *MMWR Morb Mortal Wkly Rep* 47:326–31.

Stansfeld, S.A., et al. 1998. Psychosocial work characteristics and social support as predictors of SF-36 health functioning: The Whitehall II Study. *Psychosom Med* 60:247–55.

Weight

Bender, R., et al. 1998. Assessment of excess mortality in obesity. *Am J Epidemiol* 147:42–48.

Harris, T.B., et al. 1997. Cohort study of effect of being overweight and change in weight on risk of coronary heart disease in old age. *BMJ* 314:1791–94.

Hill, J.O., and J.C. Peters. 1998. Environmental contributions to the obesity epidemic. *Science* 280:1371–73.

Jousilahti, P., et al. 1996. Body weight, cardiovascular risk factors, and coronary mortality. 15-year follow-up of middle-aged men and women in eastern Finland. *Circulation* 93:1372–79.

Kahn, H.S., et al. 1997. Stable behaviors associated with adults' 10-year change in body mass index and likelihood of gain at the waist. *Am J Public Health* 87:747–54.

Karason, K., et al. 1997. Effects of obesity and weight loss on left ventricular mass and relative wall thickness: Survey and intervention study. *BMJ* 315:912–17.

Klem, M.L., et al. 1997. A descriptive study of individuals successful at long-term maintenance of substantial weight loss. *Am J Clin Nutr* 66:239–46.

Kuczmarski, R.J., et al. 1994. Increasing prevalence of overweight among US adults. The National Health and Nutrition Examination Surveys, 1960 to 1991. *JAMA* 272:205–11.

Lean, M.E.J., et al. 1998. Impairment of health and quality of life in people with large waist circumference. *Lancet* 351:853–56.

Lee, I.M., et al. 1993. Body weight and mortality: A 27-year follow-up of middle-aged men. *JAMA* 270:2823–28.

Leibel, R.L., et al. 1995. Changes in energy expenditure resulting from altered body weight. *N Engl J Med* 332:621–28.

Means, L.W., et al. 1993. Mid-life onset of dietary restriction extends life and prolongs cognitive functioning. *Physiol Behav* 54:503–8.

National Task Force on the Prevention and Treatment of Obesity. 1994. Weight cycling. *JAMA* 272:1196–202.

Obesity: A risk factor for cardiovascular disease. 1997. *Can Med Assoc J* 157 (1 suppl).

Wing, R.R., et al. 1992. Change in waist-hip ratio with weight loss and its association with change in cardiovascular risk factors. *Am J Clin Nutr* 55:1086–92.

CHAPTER 8

Acetaminophen, NSAIDs and alcohol. 1996. *Med Lett Drugs Ther* 38:55–56.

Allison, J.E., et al. 1996. A comparison of fecal occult-blood tests for colorectal-cancer screening. *N Engl J Med* 334:155–59.

American College of Physicians. 1997. Suggested technique for fecal occult blood testing and interpretation in colorectal cancer screening. *Ann Intern Med* 126:808–10.

Bates, D.W., et al. 1995. Incidence of adverse drug events and potential adverse drug events. Implications for prevention. ADE Prevention Study Group. *JAMA* 274:29–43.

Baumeister, R.F., et al. 1995. The need to belong: Desire for interpersonal attachments as a fundamental human motivation. Review. *Psychol Bull* 117:497–529.

Cantor, K.B., et al. 1998. Drinking water source and chlorination byproducts. I. Risk of bladder cancer. *Epidemiology* 9:21–35.

Cockburn, J., and S. Pit. 1997. Prescribing behaviour in clinical practice: Patients' expectations and doctors' perceptions of patients' expectations—a questionnaire study. *BMJ* 315:520–25.

Grapefruit juice interactions with drugs. 1995. *Med Lett Drugs Ther* 37:73–74.

Hamm, R., et al. 1996. Antibiotics and respiratory infections: Are patients more satisfied when expectations are met? *J Fam Pract* 43:56–62.

Hawton, K., et al. 1994. Sexual function in a community sample of middle-aged women with partners: Effects of age, marital, socioeconomic, psychiatric, gynecological, and menopausal factors. *Arch Sex Behav* 4:375–95.

Kirkup, L., et al. 1998. Three methods compared for detecting the onset of alpha wave synchronization following eye closure. *Physiol Meas* 19:213–24.

Kronborg, O., et al. 1996. Randomised study of screening for colorectal cancer with faecal-occult-blood test. *Lancet* 348:1467–62.

Langmen, M.J.S., et al. 1994. Risks of bleeding peptic ulcer associated with individual non-steroidal anti-inflammatory drugs. *Lancet* 343:1051–52, 1075–78.

Lantz, P.M., et al. 1998. Socioeconomic factors, health behaviors, and mortality: Results from a nationally representative prospective study of US adults. *JAMA* 279:1703–8.

Lazarou, J., et al. 1998. Incidence of adverse drug reactions in hospitalized patients: A meta-analysis of prospective studies. *JAMA* 279:1200–1205.

Luckmann, R., and S.K. Melville. 1995. Periodic health evaluation of adults: A survey of family physicians. *J Fam Pract* 40:547–54.

MacDonald, T.M., et al. 1997. Association of upper gastrointestinal toxicity of non-steroidal anti-inflammatory drugs with continued exposure: Cohort study. *BMJ* 315:1333–37.

Mandel, J.S., et al. 1993. Reducing mortality from colorectal cancer by screening for fecal occult blood. Minnesota Colon Cancer Control Study. *N Engl J Med* 328:1365–71.

Muller, A.D., and A. Sonnenberg. 1995. Protection by endoscopy against death from colorectal cancer. A case-control study among veterans. *Arch Intern Med* 155:1741–48.

Murray S., et al. 1996. The self-fulfilling nature of positive illusions in romantic relationships: Love is not blind, but prescient. *J Pers Soc Psychol* 71:1155–80.

Pertschuk, M., et al. 1994. Men's bodies—The survey. *Psychology Today* 35, November/December, 35–36, 39, 72.

Sakamoto, M.S., et al. 1994. Screening flexible sigmoidoscopy in a low-risk, highly screened population. *J Fam Pract* 38:245–48.

Schiffman, S.S., et al. 1995. Effect of pleasant odors on mood of males at midlife: Comparison of African-American and European-American men. *Brain Res Bull* 36:31–37.

Schulz, R., et al. 1996. Pessimism, age, and cancer mortality. *Psychol Aging* 11:304–9.

Schwartz, J.E., et al. 1995. Sociodemographic and psychosocial factors in childhood as predictors of adult mortality. *Am J Public Health* 85:1237–45.

Smith, G.D., et al. 1996. "I'm all right, John": Voting patterns and mortality in England and Wales, 1981–92. *BMJ* 313:1573.

Smith, G.D., et al. 1998. Adverse socioeconomic conditions in childhood and cause-specific mortality: Prospective observational study. *BMJ* 316:1631–35.

Strawbridge, W.J., et al. 1997. Frequent attendance at religious services and mortality over 28 years. *Am J Public Health* 87:957–61.

Tamblyn, R., et al. 1997. Unnecessary prescribing of NSAIDs and the management of NSAID-related gastropathy in medical practice. *Ann Intern Med* 127:429-38.

Tucker, J.S., et al. 1996. Marital history at midlife as a predictor of longevity: Alternative explanations to the protective effect of marriage. *Health Psychol* 15:94–101.

Vandenbroucke, J.P. 1998. Maternal inheritance of longevity. *Lancet* 351:1064.

Wannamethee, S.G. 1996. Influence of fathers' social class on cardiovascular disease in middle-aged men. *Lancet* 348:1259–63.

Whiteman, M.C., et al. 1997. Submissiveness and protection from coronary heart disease in the general population: Edinburgh Artery Study. *Lancet* 350:541–45.

Index